THE GUYS' GUIDE TO **BEING A**

BIRTH
PARTNER

THE GUYS' GUIDE TO **BEING A**
BIRTH PARTNER

Andrew Shaw

Everything You Need
to Plan for Birth and
Bring Your Baby Home

**ROCKRIDGE
PRESS**

Interior and Cover Designer: Richard Tapp
Art Producer: Samantha Ulban
Editor: Rochelle Torke
Production Editor: Emily Sheehan

Illustrations © Caroline Attia , 2020

ISBN: Print 978-1-64739-726-5 | eBook 978-1-64739-429-5
R0

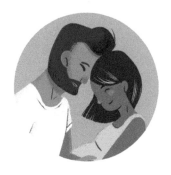

DEDICATION

To my ever-supportive, ever-understanding, and ever-compassionate wife. You're a wonder to me. To my kids, Elliott, Quinn, and Hannah, who inspire me to want to help other dads feel as special as you make me feel. To my parents and to my in-laws who have done so much, past and present, to help take care of me and my family. And finally, this book is dedicated to you, new dad. You're going to do amazing things as a father. I'm proud to be a small part of that journey.

Contents

Prologue

"You don't know what you don't know" may be the most appropriate description of childbirth.

My wife's due date for our firstborn was still a few weeks away when the contractions started. Soon we found ourselves in a hospital room where Sara could be monitored. Everything was going smoothly, aside from the small fact that we were well ahead of schedule and Sara's parents were out of state instead of with us. We watched a Harry Potter movie, her favorite, as a distraction.

I held her hand as the contractions progressed and labor got very, very real while she received an epidural. We tried to tap into our childbirth classes and our carefully considered birth plan. We tried to keep level heads and calm nerves. We both wanted to see into the future, to see how it would all unfold. But birth is more mysterious than that.

You don't know if labor will take hours and hours or if your baby will slide out like a slippery little fish. You know your whole life is about to change, but you don't know exactly how.

You don't know that your heart can handle so much more love—and then it does.

There's a lot you don't know when you become a new parent.

I'm now three kids in. My son, Elliott, is in grade school and our twin daughters, Quinn and Hannah, are just two years behind him. They were born at 31 weeks and needed extensive time in the neonatal intensive care unit (NICU)—yet another "you don't know" scenario.

However, as you head into this extraordinary unknown, there's a lot of knowledge you can gather now and take with you for the big arrival. That's where this book comes in. I've written it with dads like me in mind, as preparation for the intense-yet-magical period right before delivery, through birth, and into the first days with your new baby. It should help you ask great questions, be patient, and help you give your best to your partner and your family.

I hope this book prepares you for upcoming doctor visits and conversations with your partner about how she wants to approach childbirth. You'll be making a lot of decisions, big and small, and this book will help you understand what everyone is talking about beforehand. Involved fatherhood starts right now, and I congratulate you for it.

I'm here to help you in these pages and through my blog at InstaFather.com. Read, ask questions, have honest conversations with your partner, and let me know how it goes.

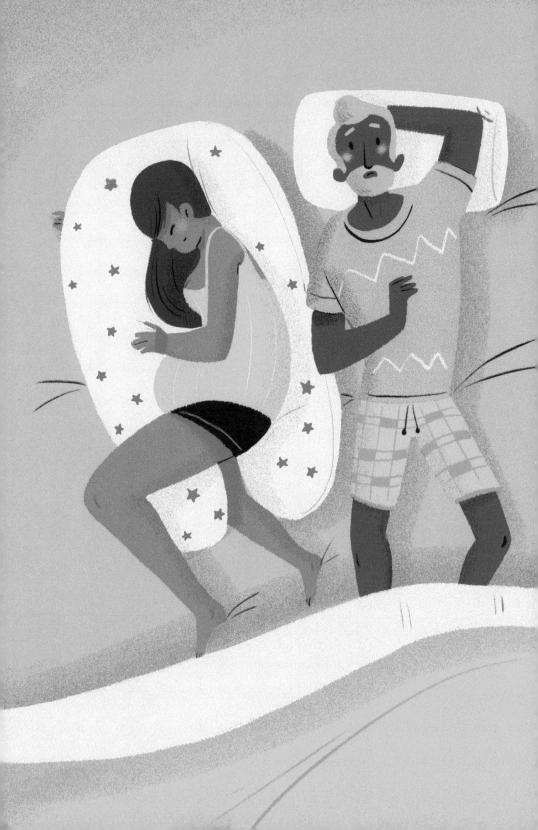

CHAPTER ONE

THE THIRD TRIMESTER: FINAL COUNTDOWN

Congratulations! You and your partner are on your way to parenthood. As a dad, you're not experiencing all the physical highs and lows of pregnancy, but you've been at your partner's side. You're sharing the journey even if you might sometimes feel like the copilot. You might even be thinking, "It'll be so nice once the baby is here. Then we'll be done with pregnancy and it will just be smooth sailing."

Well, I have some good news and I have some *interesting* news.

The good news is that you are mere weeks away—full term is 37 weeks, with most women going into labor by week 42—from meeting your little son or daughter. It's an unbelievable experience—a miracle, in fact. As a father of three, I can tell you for sure that you're going to hit a whole new level of love.

The interesting news is that birth is an adventure, and like all good adventures, you can prepare for it, you can be thrilled about it or terrified of it, but you can't write the whole story by yourself. You can't control everything about birth, but you can show up with knowledge, a calm and open mind, and a great attitude. Will you and your partner be able to handle it? Yes. But I like to be candid with new parents: The best thing you can do right now is enjoy these final few weeks with the bun inside while preparing for the day when that oven door pops open.

Now for more good news! That preparation is laid out for you in this book. And it all starts with thinking about your birth plan.

CREATING A BIRTH PLAN

One of the smartest shared activities you can do before your baby arrives—other than taking a nap—is creating a birth plan. This can be a game changer. You wouldn't send a team onto the field without plays drawn up, even if they may only be audible at the line of scrimmage. A birth plan is the same thing. It's a written plan for the birth you'd like to have in an ideal world. Couples generally write a birth plan to capture all their preferences around the big day so they don't blank on anything important in the heat of the moment.

This plan can help you set an agenda as you talk to doctors, nurses, midwives, doulas, family members—anyone and everyone on your birth team—about your wishes and goals for the birth. It may also be helpful as you decide on the kinds of medical interventions you prefer or wish to avoid. The birth plan can be as simple or detailed as you both want it to be.

You may have worked on this well in advance, perhaps after going through a childbirth class together. If you haven't started on a plan yet, there's still time as long as the baby is still inside.

Even if you only refer to the plan once or twice on delivery day, it'll be worth your time, if only to serve as a conversation starter with your partner. You don't want to find out when she's eight centimeters dilated that she has no intention of having anyone in the delivery room other than the doctor and a nurse. (Sorry, Grandma.) She may want an epidural, but you figured she'd go all natural (something you should leave up to her, by the way).

The more knowledgeable you are in advance about your options, the more you can be an advocate for your partner. That's what a dad's role in childbirth comes down to: You are your partner's and your baby's best advocate.

You can be the calm and confident voice your family needs. And with the plan in your hand, you know that what you are advocating for is in line with her needs and wants. There's no need to second-guess. This may also reassure your partner when or if she feels like she is losing control.

Before she starts pushing, there's a whirlwind of activity—and you want to focus on your partner, not on frantically trying to remember what Pitocin does.

However, keep in mind that a birth plan, no matter how well thought out, is a suggested guide. It cannot be concrete. The medical staff should be open to reviewing it with you, but it won't be their guiding blueprint. Be flexible. If it's an emergency situation, you may not get the scented-candles-and-mood-music variety of childbirth. The medical team's first and only priority is keeping everyone healthy.

What do you need to know in order to make a plan? We're going to cover that throughout this book.

After reading this book and doing any additional research that has been inspired by it, you'll be able to sit down with your partner and write down your answers to questions like these:

The Basics: Who, Where, and How

» Who would you like to include on your birth team?

» Where would you like the birth to happen (home, birth center, hospital)?

» Do you plan to have a doula or a birth attendant of your choice assist the birth?

» Do you wish to have a midwife present at the birth, regardless of the location?

» Are medical students allowed to help?

» What's your planned delivery method? (vaginal, C-section, water birth)

» Are family and friends allowed in the room during the birth?

>> How soon would you like to welcome visitors?

>> Would your partner like photos or video of the birth or no cameras allowed?

Pain Management Considerations

>> What kind of pain management techniques have you researched and found interesting?

>> Would you like to explore and use techniques such as Lamaze, Bradley Method, hypnobirthing, or acupressure?

>> Would you like to have a water tub or bathtub available?

>> Have you discussed the pros and cons of getting an epidural? How does your partner feel about this intervention?

>> What about urinary catheters or an IV? (needed if she's getting an epidural)

Comfort

>> Do you want music playing? Do you want the room as quiet as possible?

>> Does she have a birthing position that she prefers, or would she like to find the most comfortable one at the time if possible? Some women prefer to stand or squat, while others lie on their backs. There are options such as birthing tubs as well.

>> Does she want to wear her own clothes? (My wife had her own custom hospital gown to feel a little more comfortable.)

>> Does she have any dietary restrictions?

» How would you like pain relief handled?

» Do you want to catch the baby?

Unexpected Events

» What are you okay with if the delivery isn't progressing as planned? (This can be called labor augmentation, such as membrane stripping.)

» How does your partner feel about Pitocin, a drug used to induce and speed up contractions?

» Does your partner want a health provider to break the bag of waters if it doesn't happen naturally?

» What is your preferred course of action if the baby is in the breech position? Would you like staff to try to rotate him or her first before taking more drastic measures?

» What is your position on forceps or vacuum-assisted birth if the baby is stuck?

» Do you have a stance on getting a C-section? Is it only for an emergency?

» If the baby or the mom's life is at risk, do you have an idea what you'd like done?

» In the event of an emergency, which family members should be contacted by your birth team? Go ahead and capture their contact info just in case others need to reach them on your behalf.

» If the baby needs to go to the NICU, do you want one or both of you to immediately go with the child?

After the Baby Is Out

» Would you like to cut the cord? (I recommend it.)

» Do you want to keep the placenta? (Some moms freeze-dry it and consume it for the nutrients. It might sound crazy. But then again, is it?)

» Are you planning to save the cord blood? (Some families do because of stem cells in the cord blood that can be used to treat diseases.)

» Do you want to be able to hold your baby immediately with skin-to-skin contact? (Many new parents choose to do this to bond with the child right away—and dads can do it, too.)

» Do you want to stay with the baby for whatever procedures he or she needs?

» Does your partner want to try to breastfeed right away?

» Do you want to help with the baby's first bath?

» If it's a boy, do you want a circumcision? (This topic is worth researching. We opted to skip this procedure after seeing minimal medical justification and some reasons for concern regarding side effects. More and more parents of baby boys are opting out.)

Writing a birth plan gives you a chance to arm yourself with knowledge and dream of your best-case scenario while preparing for challenges or detours in advance. In this way, it's both a joyful and slightly comforting activity. Do give it serious thought. It's important for both of you to talk about your vision while also preparing to accept the birth as it unfolds. The birth plan is a great shared step toward welcoming your little one into the world in a way that feels right for both of you.

Mother and Baby in the Home Stretch at Eight Months

Is your partner giving birth to a baby or a fruit salad? You may assume it's the latter, as you've likely heard the OB-GYN describe your baby as a grape, an orange, and any number of other fruits. At eight months—in the 29- to 35-week range, or the middle of the third trimester—your baby is somewhere between a coconut and a pineapple in size. At this point, your baby begins to detect light and practice breathing.

Your partner, meanwhile, is just starting to hit the "Get this baby out of me!" stage as the fetus is rapidly gaining weight and making his or her presence known.

This period is a fantastic opportunity for you to step up. It's a chance to show Mom that you're going to be the kind of dad your baby needs—a job that begins before delivery day. Be empathetic if she needs to vent about her physical journey. Be proactive in getting her help or medicine.

Some potential issues:

Hemorrhoids: Blood flow is getting restricted down low, and that can lead to painful veins in her backside.

> ▸ **Action step:** Warm baths and ice packs can help. Asking "How are those hemorrhoids doing?" will not.

Frequent urination: It may seem like a pregnancy movie trope, but it's true. That little fella is sitting on your partner's bladder.

▸ **Action step:** Be understanding if an extra rest stop (or three) is needed. She can't help it, and rolling your eyes will not be appreciated.

Fatigue: Think of what would happen if you had to grow a human on top of the energy you already expend during the day. Feeling exhausted is, more than likely, inevitable.

▸ **Action step:** Without her having to ask, give her time to nap by running errands that she would normally do. Rearrange your schedule if need be. She probably won't say no to a preestablished break.

Swelling: Her fingers, face, and ankles may swell, which is normal.

▸ **Action step:** She may enjoy foot massages, or you could put on music and gently encourage a relaxing activity like a bath. If major swelling occurs, call the doctor, as this can be a sign of preeclampsia, a dangerous condition.

Stress: Things are getting very real for her. It's natural for her to feel worried or anxious, especially if this is her first baby or if there have been complications.

▸ **Action step:** Preparation matters. The more informed you are as a team, such as by attending childbirth classes, the more in control you both may feel. She needs to feel like you're in this together. Hopefully, she won't feel as though she has to bother you to get involved.

CHOOSING THE BIRTH LOCATION AND TEAM

Where should you have your baby? The obvious answer may be your local hospital, but for many new parents, there are alternatives that may be a better fit. I know friends who have had wonderful home births, for example. Many others have involved a doula to have a supportive expert on hand.

My partner and I decided to go the hospital route. Luckily, we were blessed to have had a viable local option with a first-class NICU when our twins were born. How did we know this was the best option for us? We took a tour and asked questions. You can contact the hospital to schedule a tour and use that time to evaluate the hospital firsthand.

What should you look out for?

Birth Plan Attitudes

You don't have to wait to see how your birth plan will be accommodated. Ask the staff during the hospital or birthing room tour; it should be apparent how they view birth plans. While you can't expect them to guarantee 100 percent adherence to your birth plan, it's good to know if they are open to reviewing it beforehand. You don't want to be blindsided on delivery day if they scoff at your requests and lean into their own protocol. Some hospitals will tell you if they are comfortable with natural birth, for example. Others will tell you that you'll be "going against the grain" if you'd like to have a natural birth at their facility.

Doctors have varying degrees of comfort with natural birth and their training is typically focused on how to administer interventions or respond to emergencies.

Midwives

These are specially trained birthing experts; midwives are medically trained and focus on delivering a baby using minimal interventions. Note that midwives can't administer an epidural or perform a C-section, but they are highly skilled at other interventions and managing common birth hiccups such as breech babies, back labor, or stalled labor. They're also well versed in different birth positions and natural pain management strategies.

Doulas

Doulas are trained birth support professionals. They focus more on the wellness of the mother. Doulas can also help you find your role as a supportive dad, too. Having a midwife on staff indicates the hospital supports natural, vaginal birth. The presence of either a midwife or doula is a positive sign that the hospital encourages moms to have support on hand.

Lactation Support

Breastfeeding can be a beautiful experience. However, for many new moms, it is also a challenging one. Does the hospital have lactation consultants who specialize in helping with breastfeeding? We used our hospital's consultants for our son, and they were incredibly supportive of my wife and empathetic with the early challenges.

Skin-to-Skin Contact

Are parents allowed to immediately hold their newborn skin-to-skin, or does the hospital prefer to wait a certain period? Dads can instantly bond with the baby by doing this and some research indicates that it's helpful to the baby's nervous system to be held against the skin, feeling the heartbeat of a care provider, immediately after birth. For my wife, holding our babies, even for a minute, right after birth was an overwhelming moment of joy.

Length of Stay

Does the hospital allow moms to rest and recuperate overnight? Or do they send them out the same day? Check with your insurance carrier as well. Speaking of which . . .

Insurance Coverage

Does your insurance work with this hospital? Are there restrictions? You don't want to be surprised or have to worry in the heat of the moment if you can afford some aspect of care.

Are you considering the home birth route? This can be an excellent option. However, if your partner has any preexisting conditions or if this is a high-risk pregnancy, your doctor will need to advise you on whether this is a viable option. If home birth is the plan, you will need to interview independent midwives who specialize in home birth.

Since not all pregnancies are ideal for a home birth, such as multiples or if she's had a previous C-section, please consult your doctor before making this decision concrete. If your partner feels strongly about having one, it helps to know that home births are safe and have a lower rate of deliveries ending in a C-section than those in a hospital. A home birth can also be ideal if your partner wants to try a natural birth (minimal or no drugs for pain or induction); if she wants to be in a familiar setting; if she has religious/cultural reasons; if a medical setting isn't nearby; or if she wants more control over how her childbirth happens. Cost can be a factor as well.

Worried that your baby could be at risk without a hospital surrounding you? As long as she's discussed a plan with her doctor and has a trained professional on hand, such as a midwife, there's every reason to think she can have a beautiful home birth experience. If the baby seems in distress or something doesn't go according to plan, make a plan for how you will take her to the hospital. Contact her doctor when she goes into labor so that medical staff are prepared in case the need arises.

My wife and I did not choose the home birth route simply because the decision seemed outside of our control. Since my wife had a high-risk pregnancy (blood clotting) and then multiples, our doctor advised us that the hospital was a safer route. I'd like to think she would have rocked a home birth, if given the chance. If your partner is interested, remember that she's the one delivering a baby. Of course, it's important to give each other's wishes serious consideration. Again, also check with your insurance. Some plans have gray areas, and this is not a time for surprises.

You can rent a birth tub, as well as other items for home births, to make your place a labor and delivery oasis. If you get a midwife, see if they have been certified by the American Midwifery Certification Board.

PLANNING AHEAD FOR PAIN MANAGEMENT

"Give me the drugs!"

Any sitcom with a pregnant woman in labor seems to have that line. You may have already imagined what your partner will sound like as she's giving birth, weeks before the due date. Wherever the birth happens, comfort management is essential to talk over with your partner, sooner rather than later.

Still, don't assume your partner is going to have to scream at a nurse while crushing your hand and swearing at you for "doing this to me!"

In fact, she may not need heavy doses of medication at all. Every birth is different and thinking through potential scenarios can help. The position of the baby, for example, can be a big factor in how strenuous labor is, and so is the size of your kiddo.

You won't find many moms who say that labor was like going to a day spa. However, don't assume every mom experienced the seventh circle of hell either. Believe it or not, some moms report feeling only "pressure" or mild discomfort during birth.

Just remember one very important thing when labor finally arrives: She's the one pushing a baby out. If she wants medication, this is her choice. You are an involved, awesome dad and your partner's greatest advocate. You are right by her side, but you can't know how she feels. It's a smart idea to talk well in advance about what kind of medication she feels is acceptable. Her feelings may change in the moment, so your job is to know the plan, then be flexible. The doctor might also decide that under certain circumstances—such as a slow fetal heart rate—pain medication needs to be reduced or avoided.

So, what are some potential pain management options?

First off, there are approaches to labor to help lessen pain without medication. Lamaze, for example, increases relaxation in your partner while you help massage and keep her occupied. Your childbirth class may also teach the Bradley Method, a relaxation approach that has your partner focus on tuning in to her body with your support. Others have benefited from hypnobirthing, breath work, water birth, and acupuncture or acupressure. Note that natural pain reduction strategies are numerous, but they're typically something you'll need to explore on your own and then bring that knowledge with you to the hospital, if you're having a hospital birth. The time to learn hypnobirthing techniques, for example, is well before the big event.

Even if your partner opts for an epidural, she will still need your full attention and support. Based on my wife's experience, this pain blocking procedure can actually be quite unpleasant when administered. Other women find it to be a godsend that makes all the difference in minimizing pain. It's important to note that there is a point of no return for epidurals, based on how far along labor has progressed. It's possible that the labor is moving so rapidly that there is no time; an epidural can take up to 15 to 20 minutes to take effect. For our twins, the epidural hadn't kicked in when they started to come out. However, she said that for our son's birth, "it worked great!"

If your partner chooses an epidural, she will initially get a local anesthetic to numb the area (near the base of her spine) before getting a larger needle with the heavy stuff. This should alleviate much of the pain so that your partner mostly feels pressure; this helps her know how hard to push. If your partner is getting a C-section, she may instead get a spinal block.

Opioids may be available to ease pain but will not numb the body and may affect the baby. These drugs may make your partner feel sleepy, but they can help to lessen pain if the labor is lasting many hours.

It's important to have your birth plan outline your partner's preferences for pain management. This helps the medical staff anticipate how to assist. And yes, plans change. Maybe you both hope to have a natural birth—and then things get real and she changes her mind. Flexibility and acceptance are two keys to a positive birth experience.

Late-Stage Tests

By this point, your partner and her OB-GYN are seeing each other regularly. If the pregnancy is high-risk, there are probably doctor checkups every week. My wife, for example, has a blood clotting disorder that required regular ultrasounds. We actually loved the extra glimpses.

Attending doctor's visits is one way to get involved before your baby arrives. If work or other obligations prevent you from going, below is a list of potential tests and screenings that will likely be offered in the third trimester. This way, at least you will know what in the GBS is happening (Group B Streptococcus—see, you're learning!).

Tests may include:

Fetal heart monitoring: This is a primary way to see how your baby is doing throughout the pregnancy.

Group B strep test: This is done between her 35th and 37th weeks of pregnancy. The doctor is checking for a GBS infection. This usually isn't a big deal for the mom but can cause serious problems for a newborn if left untreated.

Nonstress test: If you both took a nonstress test as new parents, trust me, you'd fail. But your baby? The doctor is checking for responses to stimulation and for oxygen levels. Maybe they should call it the "A-OK" test.

Stress test: During this test, the doctor is checking the fetal heart rate response to simulated contractions to see how prepared the baby is for labor.

Paternity test: Just kidding. But hey, no judgment.

PREPPING YOUR HOME FOR BABY

Your home may already be overwhelmed with baby gear. How much of this stuff do you need right away? Honestly, almost none of it—at least not right away and all at once.

Your newborn can't move yet, so the baby-proof handles and corner bumpers won't be of any use right now. She can't hold her head up, so there goes the bouncer. And he doesn't walk, so why do baby shoes even exist? Well, actually, they are adorable and that's the real point, right?

Basic Gear for Baby

A great way to help prepare for birth and parenting a newborn is by helping your partner create safe and sanitary spaces in your home for relaxing and playing with your baby. Many couples create a few convenient spaces around the home. For example, put together the crib in the nursery, place a bassinet by your bed, and/or a pack 'n play with a changing pad in the living room. You don't need a nursery if you don't have the space for it; in the same light, if you can make a nursery, enjoy making it cozy for all of you. All your baby really needs is your attention and love. Seriously. Below is a list of items to purchase in advance and keep around the house:

Crib: No soft blankets. No puffy crib bumpers. No pillows. It all can look nice, but they can create suffocation hazards. Think "bare is best." The crib itself needs to be up to code; a hand-me-down may have slats too far apart, for example. I know this can all seem overly dramatic, but your newborn is relying entirely on you at this point. It's worth being cautious.

Changing station: Stock with newborn-size diapers, wipes, diaper rash cream, and a place to put dirty diapers. We started out with a Diaper Genie but eventually just reused plastic grocery bags. An antimicrobial mat is a good spot for changing. Oh, and as much hand sanitizer as possible. Maybe just drink it with your morning coffee.

Bassinet: If your partner plans on nursing at night, it helps to have a safe, flat place to put the baby in your bedroom that is not in your bed. The merits and dangers of co-sleeping with your baby are worth researching as they get older. When it comes to a newborn, most research advocates giving the baby his or her own bed as a safer choice. Co-sleeper cribs are another option, as they can be placed directly beside the bed. This can all make life easier, especially when it's the middle of the night and you're both too tired to think straight. True story: I was once so sleep-deprived as a new dad that I woke up in a panic, sure that I had fallen asleep with our son under the covers of our bed. I riffled through the blankets only to realize I had put him back in his crib where he was safely sleeping soundly. Parenting is weird.

Swaddle blankets: Swaddling can help your baby feel secure (and thus less likely to cry). This is definitely a skill that requires practice. Use a teddy bear if you need to, but up your swaddle game before the baby arrives. Try swaddling your partner? You never know; maybe she'll find it soothing.

Stroller: Some will work with your car seat so you can simply click the seat in and be on your way. Do not feel like you need to splurge for some fancy stroller that has shocks and Wi-Fi and a water feature. It just needs to do the job and, perhaps most important, fold easily. If you think you may take long walks or exercise with your baby, a jogging stroller can help. Really, the stroller's most important role is getting you out of the house.

Mission Critical: The Car Seat

Don't be that guy who forgets the car seat. You won't be able to take your baby home without it and yes, someone from the hospital does walk out and check your car to confirm it's there and installed properly. Have it preinstalled in the car well before the due date—just in case. Since many people don't do it right the first time, police departments and other organizations often have special days when they will check your car seat installation for free. For example, newborns are rear-facing, which might not be your first guess.

Car seats can become the bane of your existence. However, some models are more user-friendly than others. Infant car seats click into a base, which makes it easier to pop them in and out. Many new cars have LATCH hooks in between the seat cushions. These allow for an easy install of your car seat. If your vehicle doesn't have LATCH hooks, most car seat brands also allow for the use of a seat belt to install them. Just be sure that the belt can be pulled tight enough so that the seat doesn't wiggle. A little trick: Pull out the seat belt as far as it goes, making sure not to let it draw back. Loop the belt through the car seat opening and click it in. Then release the belt before tightening. Otherwise, you'll never get it tight enough. Trust me. I have sworn at many a car seat.

Remember, it is unsafe to put heavy blankets or thick coats on any child in a car seat, especially newborns. They design special covers that go over top if you are having a baby in the winter. Make sure the chest strap is above the sternum, too. Don't worry. This will all be second nature before you know it.

WHEN BABIES ARRIVE EARLY

My wife and I needed to adopt the March of Dimes mindset when our twins were born at 31 weeks—nine weeks early. They are now kindergarten age, but I remember vividly the April day they were born, which was supposed to be in June. About 1 in 10 babies is born prematurely (before 37 weeks).

Our babies tried to come out at 27 weeks, which would have been a dangerous situation, and my wife had to go on hospital bed rest for several weeks. This was a grueling experience for her as an active woman and the mom of a toddler. Bed rest is not uncommon and could be in your partner's future as a method to slow down contractions and stop dilation from increasing.

The truth is, neither of you can know for sure when your baby will be born. Due dates are best guesses, after all. Your partner may have some factors that can contribute to the likelihood that she won't be able to carry your baby to term: carrying multiples, a history of premature births, or tobacco/substance abuse. However, sometimes it just happens.

My daughters were four pounds each at birth. Combined, they were less than the weight of most solo newborns. And yet, like so many preemies, they were fighters. Aided by an incredible NICU staff, they grew to be healthy babies.

The thought of having your baby born at a size that's about the length of your thumb to your outstretched pinkie finger might send a shiver up your spine. The uncertainty of it all can be unnerving—it's not what we all think of when we imagine our newborn. Yet, premature babies who have no long-term health issues are born every day. If this is the case for you and your partner, you'll begin to get to know the medical jargon and adjust to the pace of growth. It will just become a thing you do, your family's personal story. Your partner can still breastfeed, and you can still swaddle and hold your baby. You adjust.

If your baby's first stage of life requires a stay in the NICU, you can do it. So many parents do. You may have a healthy, happy baby who just needed intense care to get started. We wouldn't have chosen the NICU, but I'm also sure that we are better parents because of it.

The rough estimate with preemies is that they'll be able to leave the hospital around their original due date. For us, that meant waiting from April 7 until June, which felt like 20 years. As with every upset in life, you adjust. You begin to focus on what your baby needs that day. We celebrated the little victories, like getting to put clothes on the babies or watching the reductions in their bradys (slow heart rates). All of a sudden, a month had passed and the end was in sight.

No book about birth partners would be complete by assuming that all births happen when and how we expect them to happen. It's not all smooth sailing for many babies. The NICU isn't a simple hospital stay, and your baby won't initially have the same milestones as a full-term baby—yet. From the outside, when all friends see is a photo of your newborn, it might be easy for them to assume you're just waiting around for the baby to come home—that at least you're "getting some rest."

This is ridiculous. In all honesty, not being able to hold your baby, and even then, with wires attached, can be upsetting. Well-meaning friends and family might be constantly asking for updates because, well, that's standard with a newborn. However, if your family is in a high-stress situation, you may decide not to share much until everyone is home or just to make brief updates. Do not feel obligated to be all smiles or go over every detail with everyone. You'll go crazy, and so will your partner. There's no rush.

Having the baby early is outside of your control. You *are* in control of being there for your newborn. That's making you a good parent before you've even left the hospital. Make friends with the staff. Ask a ton of questions. Advocate for your baby—you already have a hell of a fighter.

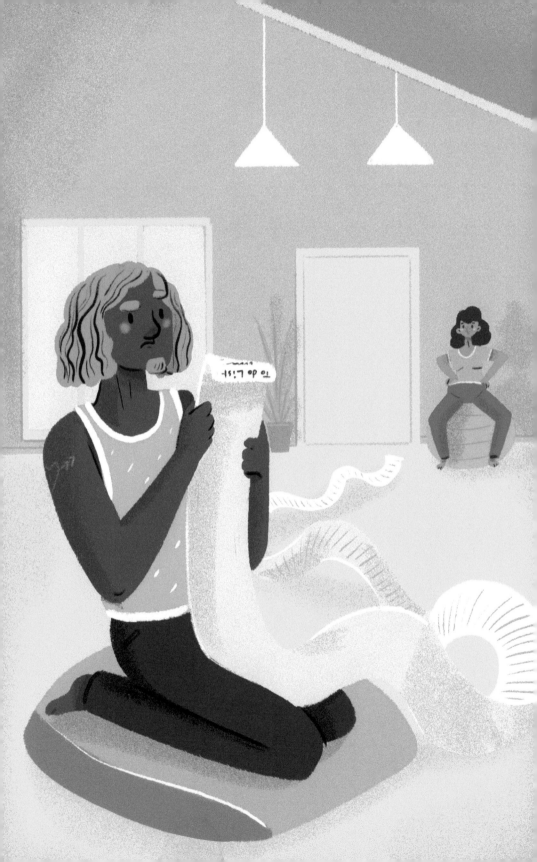

CHAPTER TWO

ANY DAY NOW

By now, you've mastered all your partner's pregnancy cravings. You've built the crib. You've taken the childbirth classes together. You looked at baby names forever and perhaps wondered why it's called "baby names" when it's the same name they'll have as an adult. You stocked up on diapers, wipes, and sanitizer—and remembered to put extras in your car. You took the dog for a walk with the empty stroller. (Seriously! It's a good way to help a dog get used to a newborn in advance.)

All you need now is a baby. Otherwise, you just look like a crazy person who can't stop talking about pack 'n plays.

Soak up these moments with your partner. You don't need me to tell you that life is going to change, but it is helpful to be reminded that this is the last time in which you can pour all your energy into just her. And she probably needs it. There's a lot on her mind.

It's important you share your emotions, too, even if that's not your style. Pregnancy does not lend itself to being rational, and in the final days before delivery, all the waiting can lead you both into emotional spirals. You may find yourself or your partner frantically googling. My wife searched for images of other mothers of multiples who were 38 weeks pregnant. Then she called me somewhat frantically to ask how her belly was ever going to stretch that far.

This isn't the time to assume she knows what you're feeling. She wants to know what emotions you have, even if the emotion is terror about becoming a dad. This is not the time to make her guess how you are feeling. More than likely, she'll be grateful for your openness and honesty.

That might seem counterintuitive. Why let her know you're nervous if you're trying to make her feel calm? Because without you being honest, she's going to feel like she's the only one freaking out. That's just going to make her even more anxious.

You can be the calm surrounding the uncertainty. If you feel this way, admit that you're nervous, but reassure her that you are there for her. Let her know you will research anything she needs. Rub her shoulders and feet and show her that you're triple-checking the hospital bag. Open up to her—and ask what she needs. You can also help both of you feel better by going back over your birth plan and practicing birthing positions.

During these last few weeks, she can continue exercising. Sex is still possible, too, if she's up for it. In fact, your doctor may even advocate for you two to have sex to stimulate labor.

PACKING FOR THE HOSPITAL

A great way to pass the time while waiting for baby is to pack your bag for the hospital. You can expect to be there from one to three nights though sometimes the stay is longer if the baby or mom needs extra support after the birth. I recommend packing with the three-day time frame in mind.

What to Pack for Mom

Toiletries: The hospital may provide some items, but you might as well make sure she's covered with a toothbrush and a basic toiletries kit.

Designer maternity gown: Optional? Hell yes. Awesome? Absolutely. My wife ordered a maternity gown that made her feel a little more comfortable and not so "blah." Why not? It made her feel more at ease when she was in labor, and that was worth it. Plus, it's cool for the photos. *Optional idea: Let her pick one out and buy it for her as a push present.*

Lotion: Good idea to have on hand for stretched or dry skin.

Essential oils: If she's into it, essential oils such as lavender can have a calming effect. I had some on my wrists so that as I helped her with delivery, she could smell it.

Blanket: Expect temperature changes! And sometimes a blanket from home can add to the comfort level. Again, this is all about comfort. If there is no special blanket, skip it; the hospital will have some.

Music: A playlist for the labor process can be a fun thing to put together. Figure out if you should bring a mini Bluetooth speaker and if you need Wi-Fi to play it. We played the Hawaiian version of "Somewhere Over the Rainbow" when my son was born, for example. Ask the hospital or birthing room about the Wi-Fi situation beforehand: Is there a password? A fee? You might have a lot of downtime waiting for the action, and Netflix might come in handy.

Snacks: Warning—some anesthesiologists forbid eating before delivery because of the risk of throwing up. Others are fine with it. Many moms, including my wife, think the benefit of having some energy for the huge physical task ahead is more important than the small chance of throwing up, but you'll want to talk to your doctor ahead of time. If it's okay, or if you want food for after, pack some things you know she'll like that don't require refrigeration. You can't assume she'll want anything from the hospital. Pregnancy, as you may have heard, has a habit of making finicky eaters.

Face wipes: To help her feel refreshed after sweating during delivery but before she's ready for a shower.

Socks with tread on them/slippers: Some hospitals provide them.

Something calming to put within eyesight: Could be a framed photo of her family or pet. It could be a religious item. Maybe a cast photo of *Real Housewives*? Whatever might make her smile a little during a stressful time that you can park somewhere in eyesight.

Phone chargers: You're going to be there a while, and basics like phone chargers are easy to forget. If you do forget, nurses have told me they have a huge collection of forgotten phone chargers in the lost and found.

Clothes to go home in: Even though the baby is out, she will likely need to wear her maternity clothes home, but at least they will be nice and fresh. Since this is usually a big picture day, many women choose their "going home" outfit well beforehand. Double-check with her that you have the right clothes in the bag.

What to Pack for Little People

Newborn clothing: Pack some clothing for your baby. You'll want to bring a few onesies as well as some soft pants or leggings, socks, long- and short-sleeved shirts, a sweater or coat, newborn hats, and a small blanket.

A gift for the older child: Some families proudly give older siblings an "I'm a big brother/sister" shirt or pack gifts for the child to give to the new sibling, which can help the older child feel involved.

What to Pack for Yourself

Camera: If you have a nice camera, it'll take much better photos than your phone will indoors. Talk with your partner ahead of time to find out what she's comfortable with. Does she want photos during the delivery process? Just afterward? Any particular moment? You can be the point person for that.

Snacks: You're going to get very hungry and might not be able to slip away to the cafeteria, so bring something for yourself.

Clothes: I didn't bring enough clothing. I had to wear essentially the same thing for three days. Don't be me.

Chargers: Same as above.

Insurance card: If you've been to the hospital before, they should have you in the system, but it's always good to be careful. Again, talk to the insurance company ahead of time if you haven't at this point.

Cash: For vending machines, coffee at a kiosk, or possibly for parking.

Mom and Baby at the Finish Line

So much continues to change with your baby when you're in the final 37-to-40-week stretch. Your baby is the size of a pumpkin or a watermelon at this point. They can now be born and thrive without medical help. Their fingers are strong enough to grasp, and your little one can even sneeze.

Now is not the time to ask your wife what it feels like to swallow a bowling ball, or laugh when her swollen feet don't fit into her shoes. It's tempting to make dad jokes but try to refrain for your own safety.

You can, though, be extra patient and helpful. Her nesting instincts—that feeling she's getting to make your home perfect for the impending arrival—may be kicking in. If it's giving her something to focus on other than heartburn and soreness, roll with it. Offer to clean an area of the house, pick up items at the store, or meet up in random parking lots to pay for consignment swap site finds.

Her hormones may be hitting new highs, too. It's crucial you separate your wife's true demeanor and personality from who she might be in a given moment. Brush things off quickly. If you wonder why she seems snippy, realize the intent of what she's saying and not how she's saying it. Hormones work differently with everyone, so your partner may be calm and centered. If she's not, just keep things in perspective.

Do you know what can make the biggest difference? Handling all the little things, especially the little things she usually takes care of. I'm not just talking about doing the laundry without her asking if that was normally her area. Try writing down grocery lists, remembering to pick up a birthday card for her aunt, or calling the dog sitter—whatever you can do so she can focus on her pregnancy, just do it.

There's also something else you can do for your partner before the baby arrives—get her a push present. The idea is you offer a gift in appreciation of all she has to do that you can't possibly experience.

Your partner has gone from not seeing her ankles anymore to experiencing hours of sweaty labor that ends in her pushing out a placenta like a slab of tableside prime rib at Texas Roadhouse . . . so yeah, you can get her a necklace if she'd like one.

Your partner deserves a tangible show of appreciation, even if money is tight. You are blessed with a baby—that's not to be mistaken with receiving a gift. It's fine to show appreciation on top of that. This doesn't have to (and shouldn't) break the bank. Maybe it's a slightly fancier diaper bag or a simple piece of jewelry. An e-reader or nice earbuds may be super useful when it comes to breastfeeding. None of this is an obligation. It's about the gesture.

IN CASE YOU FEEL DISCONNECTED

Don't be surprised if you feel a bit of a disconnect, nervous, or uncertain at this point. You're excited, sure, but you may not be feeling as emotionally bonded with your soon-to-be son or daughter as your partner is. Maybe that's worrying you.

First of all, dads don't feel the baby inside them or have hormonal changes like mothers do. There are solid physiological reasons you are feeling things differently.

Secondly, for months you've been looking at your baby as a black-and-white blob in a tiny picture. It makes sense that, for some dads-to-be, it's hard to get emotional over what appears to be a Rorschach test. For some, seeing an ultrasound has a major impact, and everything becomes real. For others, it's simply a cool moment to see some visual confirmation.

Until you see fingers moving or a face, it may not seem like a baby yet, and it may not seem like your baby until he or she comes out. That's okay, too. If you're being supportive and excited about the process, you are fine. Even if you're apprehensive, you're there for her; the key is that she feels supported.

When the baby arrives, there might be a moment that everything clicks. A moment when you think, "Oh, now I get what this is about." Guys are visual. We want to see it right in front of us. I was really excited about my son, but everything didn't really fall into place until he was born. Truthfully, it took a few months before I really felt that strong fatherhood connection.

I turned out okay. You will, too. If the disconnect lingers much longer than you feel it should, talk to a professional. This is a big life change, and everyone experiences it differently.

THE WAITING GAME

Due dates are just a reference point, not a certainty, so it's hard to know when your baby is arriving if you don't have a scheduled induction. When your partner feels her first contraction, you might expect her to say something like "It's time!" or "holy #%@*!" We've all seen those movies. However, it may feel more subtle to her than that. In the land of birth, you just never know. Her water could break in a public place, or she could be lounging at home and feel the slightest squeeze in her belly. There's not always a big signal. Your partner could simply feel some pressure or wonder if she's having indigestion. These could be contractions, but they could come and go for a while before things really get cooking.

It's not uncommon for early signs of labor to occur hours or even days before labor really takes off. There are bodily functions and other signs, though, that she can look out for:

- **Bloody show:** It's a brownish discharge that indicates her cervix is nearly ready for labor.

- **Lightening:** Your partner may experience this a few weeks to a few hours before birth (or not at all). It's when the baby's head drops down into her pelvis to get ready for delivery. She may feel the baby is positioned lower because it's easier to breathe.

- **Diarrhea:** For some women, if this is happening frequently, it can mean labor is about to start.

- **Contractions:** She should pay attention to repetitive contractions, which feel at first like someone is squeezing her abdomen. It they come at regular intervals less than 10 minutes apart, that probably means it's "go" time.

- **A baby pops out:** Uh, your partner has given birth. Every once in a while, a baby comes out very fast. But usually, time is on your side.

The underlying mechanism that is so pivotal in the birth process is the dilation of the cervix. The what of the what? The cervix is the tiny passageway at the end of the uterus. The uterus is where your baby has been growing and the cervix is kind of like the gate that has to open—or dilate, as they call it—in order for the baby to come down into the birth canal. Get used to people talking about your wife's cervix a lot. Like 87 percent more often. Basically, the dilation of her cervix is the impending blizzard and the doctor is the Weather Channel. The cervix dilating doesn't mean the baby will be born that day; it just means the childbirth process is beginning.

If the cervix begins dilating well before the due date, medications such as magnesium sulfate, and/or bed rest could be prescribed to slow everything down. Bed rest is exactly like it sounds, but far from a vacation. She'll have to stay in bed nearly all the time except maybe to use the bathroom or shower or an occasional walk down the hallway. Obviously, it can be a bit nerve-racking to stay in bed at such a busy time. Be patient and understanding.

Once that magical day (or night) comes for your baby to arrive, your first step as a couple is going to be to take a deep breath. You do not have to race to the hospital or call the midwife unless contractions are about five minutes apart. Otherwise, you'll either get sent back home or you'll do a lot more waiting in the hospital.

IS LABOR STARTING?

What will your partner feel right before going into labor? How will you know if it's really happening? What is labor and birth anyway? The answers to these questions aren't as cut and dried as we might like. So, I'm going to explain some basics here and what to watch for as you get close to the big day.

Labor is different for each person and even each pregnancy. Here's a basic overview: What we call "early labor" is generally the longest stage, and it's all about the body preparing to open up. During this phase, her cervix—again, that's the circular muscle group beneath her uterus—will be quietly (or not so quietly) opening. Early labor is the period when the cervix has dilated (opened) by about three centimeters.

The interval when the cervix continues to open from three centimeters to about seven centimeters is often referred to as "active labor." This is when contractions are coming regularly and, perhaps, intensely. At about seven centimeters, things change again, often intensifying in terms of the frequency and strength of contractions. Many call this phase "transition." Once the cervix opens to 10 centimeters, your partner will feel the urge to push. We'll cover this in more detail in the next chapter, but I wanted to give you the whole birth thing in a single, simplified nutshell for now.

Have I used the word cervix enough yet? You'll be hearing it a lot before a baby drops into your arms. That's because the essence of birth, you could say, is the relaxation and opening of the cervix. This little muscle group, and the human attached to it, needs to feel safe in order to open up, and until the cervix opens, no baby is coming out. So that's one reason you'll read so often in this book about helping your partner feel calm and supported. It's mission critical in the land of birth.

It's mind-blowing how a woman's body adjusts to make birth possible. My wife was kind enough to remind me what she felt when our son was on the way. The day before he was born, she was at work and remembers feeling "miserable" all day, but she couldn't put her finger on why.

That night, cramping—kind of like you have to poop—set in, she said. She said the feeling would go away and then come back.

"After a few times, I thought 'Oh, this is it,'" she said.

That's when she woke me up in the middle of the night to tell me it was officially happening. Being the cool cat I am, I started racing around the house, throwing stuff in a hospital bag that I was planning to pack that very next day. (Now you see why I recommend doing this early.) Being the wise woman she is, my wife had me put on the brakes for a few hours until the contractions were closer to about five minutes apart. We watched *Mad Men*. It was, all things considered, very low key.

Remember that early labor may last hours—even a day or more. Your role is to make her feel relaxed and comforted. It's important to stay calm yourself, maybe even try to have a little fun. You'll soon be busy enough with a new baby, so if you can squeeze in a nice stroll or good movie beforehand, why not?

Meanwhile, perhaps your partner wants to take a shower or bath. Turn on relaxing music. Chat with friends. Call her mom. The calmer you are, the calmer she is, and that is everything when it comes to fetal heart rate and your partner's own mental well-being.

You may assume her water will break if it's the real deal, but this is not always a reliable predictor. Water breaking means the fluid-filled amniotic sac surrounding the baby has broken and labor could happen shortly. However, it doesn't happen naturally for every birth. The water could break early or later. It's also common for the sac to break, allowing a trickle of water to come out, and then nothing much happens. Again, more waiting.

Yes, yet another movie trope that has let you down. If you watched the film *Knocked Up* for the realism, it's about as realistic as Katherine Heigl dating Seth Rogen.

Still, if your partner's water breaks or if there's vaginal bleeding, call the doctor immediately.

Braxton Hicks Contractions

You may hear about women having "false alarms" at this stage. This usually refers to Braxton Hicks contractions, which feel like an irregular tightening in her lower abdomen. The intensity can vary, which, naturally, can make it feel like the "real deal." These false labor uterine contractions are named after Dr. John Braxton Hicks, who discovered them and thought it would be a genius idea to name something after himself that will piss women off for centuries to come.

Your partner is more likely to get them if she becomes dehydrated or has been on her feet a lot. They can even last for hours. Sex can also cause Braxton Hicks contractions (the price you pay, I guess). If she feels the contractions ease by drinking water or by changing positions, that's a sign it's Braxton Hicks. Take these as an opportunity to practice breathing exercises and get a sense of what's to come.

Encourage her to get a checkup to be sure if she is uncertain. New moms are expected to know what contractions feel like without having ever experienced them. Since she doesn't want to miss all the signs and give birth in the back of a cab, being extra careful is understandable.

Normal contractions gradually get stronger, happen at regular intervals, and don't ease up. You can help her time contractions and keep track. One of the first things the medical staff will ask you is how far apart the contractions are.

OKAY, THE BABY REALLY IS COMING

If you're not with your partner, you're probably going to get a text or call. I distinctly remember where I was standing at work when I got a text from my wife that our daughters were coming, which was simply a picture of the very active contraction monitor.

Do not drive like a crazy person to the hospital. If you get pulled over or get into an accident, you're only going to be that much later. Let her know you're on your way and you're good to go. Call your doctor when you think contractions have begun. They will likely have you wait to come to the hospital until there's a certain amount of time between each contraction. If you are at home timing contractions, put on soothing music or a relaxing show while you wait.

Who Ya Gonna Call?

Plan who you want to call to inform family and friends that it's go time. This will likely fall to you so your partner can focus on her body while you alert people. I suggest waiting until you have a doctor confirm it's the real deal (unless a parent/in-law coming from out of town needs a head start).

Be Ready to Wait—Again

Remember that unless her water broke or the contractions are close together, you probably have time. You'll be at the hospital waiting or at home waiting. Some people prefer to ride the early portion out in the comfort of home before heading to the hospital. (Don't wait too long or you'll need some industrial-strength carpet cleaner.) It's not uncommon for women with contractions to be sent back home for labor to progress.

Pause and Take a Breath

Take a moment, if you can, before rushing off to the hospital. Soak it in for a second. I remember telling my wife as we pulled out of the driveway, "Babe, this is probably the last time it's just the two of us." We took a moment to appreciate it, and then we were off.

THE INS AND OUTS OF INDUCTION

In a perfect world, labor starts exactly as planned and exactly when it's needed. However, you've learned by now that pregnancy doesn't always take in account things like "plans" or "statistics" or "your office pool on delivery dates."

Your partner could even go beyond the due date. Personally, I was born about a week late, a fact my mother reminds me of to this day. It's not my fault I was 9 pounds, 11 ounces, Mom—I wasn't eating burritos in there.

It can be incredibly tough to be patient and wait for labor to start. You may have your work on standby and are worried about causing a rift with your boss. Or you may have family in town to help, but there's no baby yet. Really, you just want to meet your newborn. Patience is key. You've waited this long; a few more days won't hurt.

Her doctor, however, may decide it's time and suggest inducing (kick-starting) labor. In fact, about one in four labors are induced in some form. There may be medical reasons to induce such as a stalled labor or medical emergencies. For example, her water broke some time ago, but labor is not progressing.

Several methods may be considered to help get that labor moving along:

- **Pitocin** is a synthetic version of the hormone oxytocin. It helps stimulate contractions in the uterus, so using Pitocin gives labor an extra boost. Contractions can start within a matter of hours.

- **Cervical ripening:** This is either exactly what you think or not at all what you think. The cervix is thinned or softened with saline or synthetic prostaglandins.

- **Membrane stripping/sweeping:** The doctor hastens delivery by breaking up membranes attached to the amniotic sac as a way to cause the water to break. There is a risk of bleeding and cramping with this procedure.

- **What may not work:** Home remedies such as acupuncture, castor oil, spicy food, or pineapple. Your aunt's neighbor's cousin may have had her baby after eating kung pao chicken, but that's not exactly science.

Each of the medical induction methods carry some risk—for mom and for baby—so she'll want to talk through these options. This may sound a bit scary, but remember that with labor and delivery it's all about weighing risks and benefits. What will help your partner and your baby be in the best position for good health? Ask yourself that and you'll have your answer.

You can discuss it in advance as part of your birth plan, too. My wife took an approach of requesting that labor progress as naturally as possible for as long as possible, but she also understood the entire goal was to have a healthy baby. She was ready to adjust if that's what was needed.

You may wonder why all women don't schedule an induction if it means you get more certainty on a delivery date. After all, as long as the baby is safe, why wouldn't you? It can make sense to have a scheduled induction if she doesn't live close to a hospital, for example, or if the mom has certain health challenges. A delivery for the sake of convenience is not the point. Her body knows when it's time. The baby knows when it's ready. This isn't a dinner reservation. Induced deliveries typically require additional medical interventions, including higher C-section rates. They carry risks that you'll want to discuss with your doctor. However, they can also be the safest option for some moms and babies.

When your baby arrives, no matter how early or late or right on time, it will be part of their life story. Every baby arrives differently, but in the end, they just need to be held, loved, and comforted. The delivery date is just when they decided to introduce themselves.

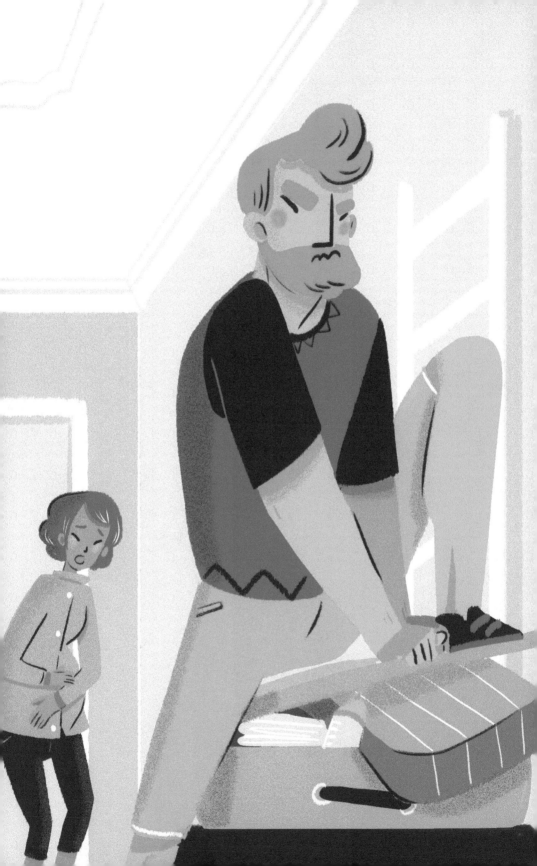

CHAPTER THREE

LABOR AND DELIVERY

Months of preparation have led to this. You are having a baby. Well, hopefully, not right this very moment because, what the heck, dude? Put down this book!

As your partner goes into labor, things can happen quickly. Or, for some women, it can take hours. The process may be "hurry up and wait" over and over again.

You may not feel ready. Bear in mind that your partner may feel the same. This is normal. You're both going to be amazing. She's going to be a rock star, and you're going to be there for every moment.

That's half the reason she's been telling you to read all those books (like this one) the past few months. It's why you have gone to at least a few OB-GYN appointments. It's why you sat through *What to Expect When You're Expecting*.

As labor progresses, you can advocate for your partner and understand what doctors and nurses are telling you. It's like your star player is in the Super Bowl and you're the coach, except instead of helping them go for a touchdown, the player is pushing a baby out. I'm assuming that would be worth more than six points.

MOVING INTO ACTIVE LABOR

As mentioned in chapter 2, the early labor stage is all about steady, regular contractions that slowly dilate her cervix to about three centimeters. Remember that the early labor phase can last up to 20 hours if it's her first pregnancy. "Can" is the key word here because for some women, it happens quickly.

Again, you don't need to rush to the hospital or call your midwife as soon as the first contraction hits. The "5-1-1" rule of thumb is easy to remember: Wait until contractions occur every five minutes, last one minute each, and have been progressing for one hour. Waiting helps in particular if she wants a low-intervention birth; she'll have fewer things administered to her if she can wait it out. (If her water broke or if she is bleeding heavily, call the doctor right away.)

The active phase of labor—anywhere from one to five hours long—occurs as she dilates from four to seven centimeters. At this point, it's critical to understand how much the mom's emotions influence birth. In fact, I think they might drive birth more than any other single factor, but I have no proof of that. Feeling calm, loved, grounded, safe, and supported are essential to allowing the cervix to relax and open. Avoid making any anxious statements, talking too much, or running around like the beheaded chicken. Try to be together calmly, enjoying the momentous reality of this time while keeping mom as comfortable as possible. This tells her nervous system (and cervix, just to throw that word at you again!) that "all is well" and that this is the perfect, safe time for having a baby. That's what the birthing mind/body needs to hear, feel, and truly believe.

At this point, the contractions will be getting stronger and closer together, which is the main sign that it's probably time to go to the hospital, birthing center, or your birthing area at home. Remember to call ahead if you're driving to a hospital so they can be ready for you and her OB-GYN can be notified. It's important to note that her doctor may not be around that day and you may end up with another physician. Most doctors want to be there for their patients, but they cannot always be available. Our babies were born with a different OB-GYN than my wife had being seeing for prenatal care. It wasn't ideal, but that's why you brought your birth plan. You did bring it . . . right?

Again, your partner is sensitive to your energy, so as much as you can, stay positive and calm. If you get frantic or frustrated, it could actually slow down the labor. That's the last thing she needs. Help her remain calm and focused. It's unlikely she needs an ambulance unless there's a true emergency. If you are taking your car, make sure your baby seat is installed. Once you arrive, the last thing you'll want to do is drive back to get it.

If you're entering a hospital, they'll get her to Labor & Delivery to start monitoring her. At home, a midwife will do likewise. It helps if you have kept track of the contractions.

Prepare for the Biggie: Transition

Now the focus is on the transition stage. This is the short, often-intense period when the cervix fully dilates, the final step before it's time to push the baby down the birth canal and out into the world. Transition can be highly uncomfortable, and this may be the time when your partner needs your calm and positivity more than ever before. If she's having a natural birth, this could be the moment when her sounds are louder as she tries to find some release for the energy in her body, and her confidence may wane.

She is feeling massive surges of sensation, and it's not time to push yet. The cervix must come to its fully open position—10 centimeters—before she can safely begin pushing. Note that the pushing will bring great relief and is generally LESS painful than the preceding stages—especially transition.

Here's what your partner will be experiencing at this critical and often-challenging phase of the birth journey:

- Her contractions are getting closer together—each can last 90 seconds and happen every two to three minutes.

- This stage lasts about 30 minutes to two hours. A pillow under her back can help.

- This may also be a great time for her to move around, soak in the birth tub, or try any method to get comfortable.

- Sometimes, it helps a woman to sit in the bathroom by herself for a few minutes, because, again, the more she can relax, the faster the cervix can open.

- The baby is moving his or her way down into her pelvis.

- She may be asking for pain medication right around now. Try the breathing exercises the two of you practiced. Let her know that it's okay to make some sound to let off the steam.

- Nausea can increase. She may feel shaky.

To help her through this, ask her what she's experiencing. "How are you feeling?" may get you a "How do you THINK I'm feeling?!" In this case, offer specific actions to help. She may say her lower back is seizing up, so you can offer to apply pressure to relieve it. She may want to try a warm bath to help ease pain, so you can get that ready. If she feels the urge to push, she should tell her doctor or midwife.

You don't have to ask her every two minutes for an update or overwhelm her with offers to do something. By doing that, you're putting the onus on her to respond to *your* need to feel involved and supportive. Do you see how that's actually counterproductive? She may only need you to listen quietly and massage her back, and if that's it, you're doing great.

There's no need to win "Childbirth Partner of the Year" every minute. No one is keeping score. You can remind her to focus on the next contraction. When she gets through one, then repeat. Soon enough, it'll be time to push.

What Not to Say in the Delivery Room

This is an intense, exciting, and life-changing time. You are there to support the mom-to-be, but it's important that you watch how you phrase things. Your partner is understandably dealing with *a lot* right now. Keep that in mind, and *do not* say the following in the delivery room:

"I'm so hungry/tired." You may be waiting awhile. It doesn't matter. Pack something in the hospital bag if need be, but no one gives a damn about how you're doing. You may have been up all night, but now is not the time to say anything.

> ▸ **What to say instead:** Nothing! Grab a coffee.

"I'd like to eat/close my eyes/do something for myself, but I don't want to leave you." This sounds like a martyr. Don't put her in a position in which she might feel guilty.

> ▸ **What to say instead:** "Do you have everything you need right now?"

"Yeah, *we* had a long night. It's been tough on *both* of us." This is not about you. It's about your partner and your baby. Don't try to steal the attention—you're not in the same category as your partner right now. Don't complain about things you're dealing with or compare the pain she feels to a sports injury you had. *It is not the same thing.*

> ▸ **What to say instead:** "She has been such a trouper all night. I can't imagine how tough this is!"

"I'm just going to turn on the game for a minute." I don't care if your favorite team is on the one-yard line about to win the Super Bowl. If your baby is on the way, you do not check out the TV or keep refreshing your SportsCenter app. You can do this if you're hoping for a divorce, I suppose. But you don't want your wife to tell your daughter one day that Daddy missed her birth because the Steelers threw an interception.

> **What to do instead:** Turn off your notifications and get someone to record the game. You can always catch up later.

"Wow! That looks like it hurts!" Of course it does, dummy. You aren't helping.

> **What to say instead:** "Give me your hand so you can squeeze."

Any jokes about blood/pooping/fluids. Just don't. You know your partner, so if you can lighten the mood to help her relax, awesome. She should be the center of attention, though. Doctors have already heard your joke a million times.

> **What to say instead:** The opposite of whatever dad joke is in your head.

CHANGING POSITIONS

Labor positions used to lack a plural. It was basically "on your back" and wait. Increasingly, women are encouraged to consider whatever position best suits them as they prepare for delivery. Many women who do not use an epidural find lying on their back extremely uncomfortable or intolerable. Positions such as crouching on all fours or standing up and leaning with their hands against a chair may feel much better. However, if she gets an epidural, the hospital may require her to stay in bed.

If she opts out of the epidural, you can gently encourage her to try different positions to get a sense of what makes her most comfortable. As the hours go by, she may decide to switch things up. Your job is to make sure she feels as supported as possible. Gently remind her to change positions frequently as labor progresses, especially if she wants to minimize drugs for pain management.

Shifting labor positions can ease her pain and keep labor moving along more quickly. The act of staying upright can help her take advantage of gravity. There is nothing saying she has to just lie back in a bed. Either way, it's her call.

Play her favorite songs, praise her like crazy, and keep mental distractions going in between contractions. Your goal is to make her feel relaxed when possible and to help ease pain and discomfort.

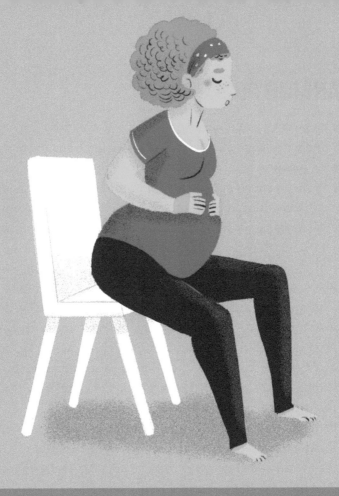

ROCKING

The gentle movement encourages that little one to keep moving down. It also helps mom's pelvis to move. She can try this either in a chair or by swaying back and forth. Ask if there's a rocking chair available. It's labor and delivery—there should be a freaking rocking chair around.

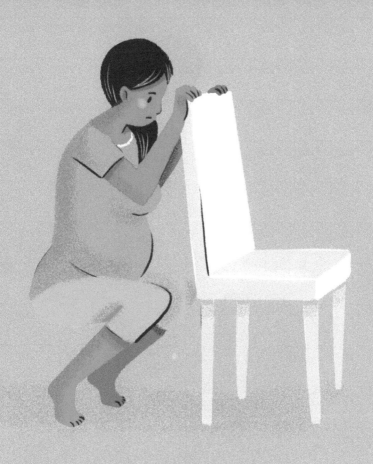

SQUATTING

This takes advantage of gravity and really opens up the pelvis. She can use this one right before or during delivery. When squatting, make sure to help her keep her balance. A birthing bar (which looks a bit like a Dance Revolution arcade platform) can also be used for support or to lean on.

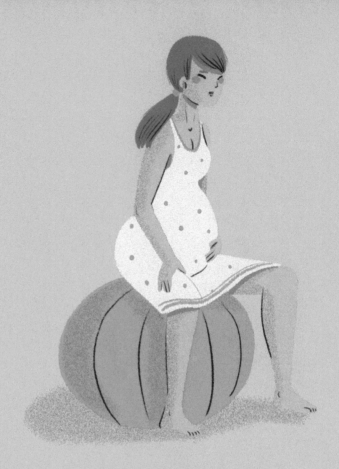

SITTING

Our hospital had birthing balls—basically, an exercise ball—available to sit on. If your partner finds that sitting upright eases contraction pain, a birthing ball can be a big help. Just be sure to watch carefully that she does not get off balance. Sitting may be less tiring than some other options. If she's in a hospital bed, you should be able to adjust it and use pillows to support her back. As a bonus, it's easy to stay close to the fetal heart machine.

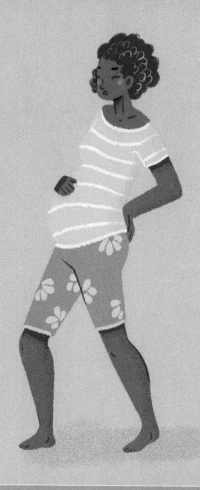

STANDING OR WALKING

When you think of a woman in labor, you don't think of her walking around, but gravity is her friend here. You can encourage her to try this earlier in labor since standing, let alone walking, will get harder as contractions ramp up. She can use this to help with backaches and reduce contraction pain as well as to move the baby down. If she wants to try to take a walk, work with nurses to make sure the fetal heart rate can still be monitored.

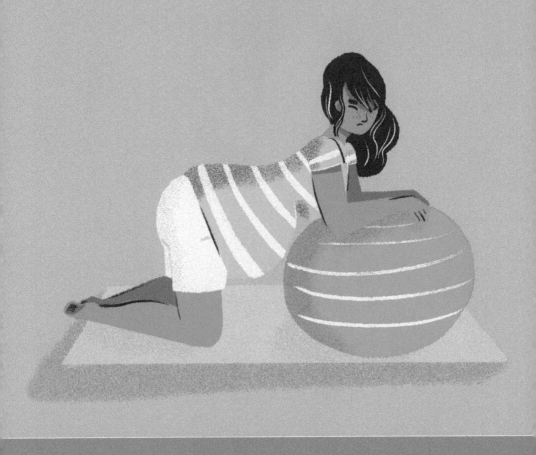

LEANING OVER OR KNEELING

You can make a small stack of pillows for her to lean on or grab the birthing ball. Why lean forward? It'll get the baby off her spine and encourage him or her to move forward. Try rubbing her back when in this position.

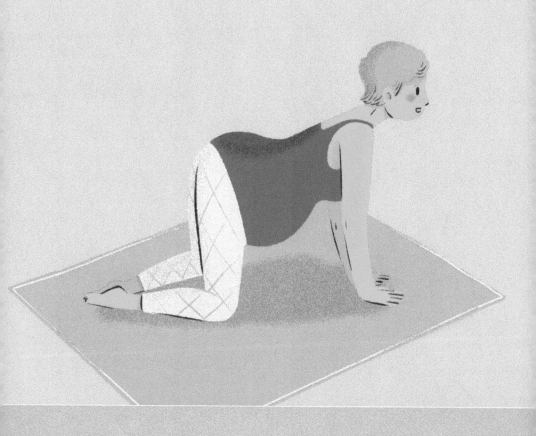

HANDS AND KNEES

Back labor is no picnic. It's a lot of pain in the lower back, and if that's the case, your partner is going to want relief. Getting on all fours can help. You can apply counterpressure to her lower back. She can even deliver in this position. Seriously. After a while, this can be tough on your partner's arms, so be ready to move her to another position, if needed.

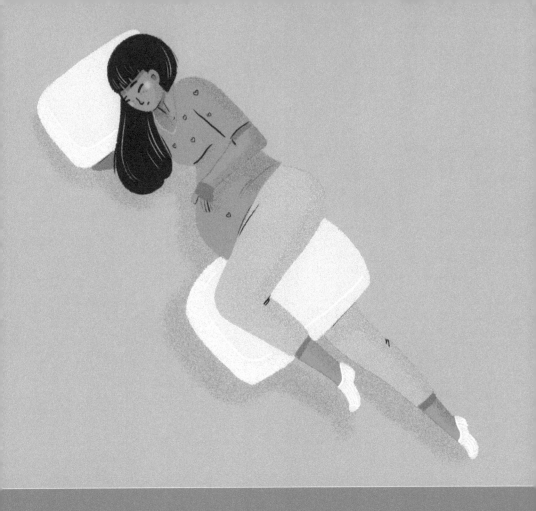

SIDE-LYING

The fetal position, in which the mother is lying on her side, can help ease contraction pain and give you some perfect massage angles. She can also rest here for a bit, which is no small thing before delivery. Depending on how the baby is positioned, it can be more difficult to track the fetal heartbeat, but the medical staff will let her know.

Breathing Techniques

There's one way to help alleviate pain during childbirth that you might not have even thought of, especially if you were unable to attend childbirth classes.

Take a deep breath and think about what's to come.

See, you're already doing it. Breathing with purpose can be highly effective. In fact, according to one survey of 2,400 mothers, breathing techniques were the most common comfort approach by women in labor, followed closely by selective amnesia. (Well, no, that was a joke. But wouldn't that be helpful?)

You can be a huge help as a breathing partner, serving as a calming influence that helps her avoid hyperventilating.

Walk her through a Lamaze approach. This involves slow, deep rhythmic breathing in the early stages of labor in a calm fashion. She can focus on you, the music, or on keeping her blood pressure down.

As she approaches the "time to push" stage, she can let out what is called an "organizing breath," or a deep sigh. With Lamaze, she will then focus deeply again on one object or person. As the contraction works its way through, she can take quick breaths followed by a long breath. This is that "hee hee hoo" you may have heard about or seen in the movies. This breathing technique uses the breath to distract her, lower stress hormones, and redirect her from focusing on the pain or fear.

During the pushing, she can take a deep breath and slowly exhale as she pushes. Remind her to take a few calming breaths after a big push. Gently remind her, that is. Remember that this is an incredible physical event, and she is being asked to perform a literal miracle with her own body. So, if she decides the breathing isn't working or that she doesn't want a reminder, that's not a problem. Go with the flow.

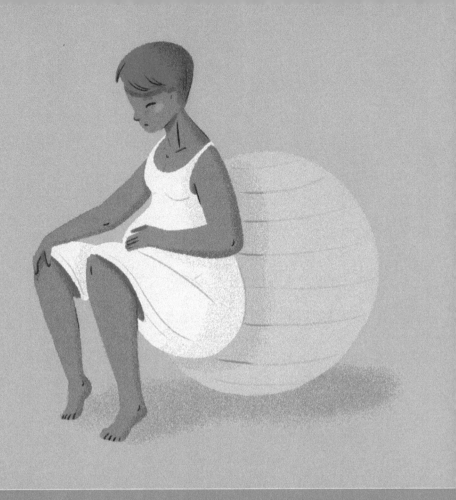

SQUATTING BIRTH POSITIONS

It makes sense when you think about it. This is how
bodies push things out. Your partner will get to use
gravity, which helps reduce the need for delivery tools
such as forceps. A birthing bar can give her something
to hold on to and push against; ask if one is available
if you don't see it in the room. Again, be sure to assist
her with balance and support. This position is a popular
approach, though it's not often talked about as part of
the birth story. Here's a fun game: Ask your mom how
she delivered you? Or maybe not. That could be a lot
of visuals.

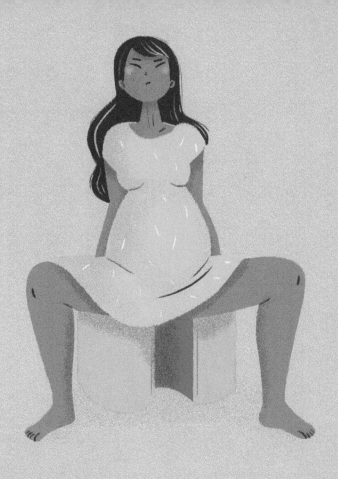

BIRTHING STOOL

A birthing stool is basically a toilet seat. That's what will pop in your head if you see it. However, it's highly effective because she can use it to squat or get on all fours and use it as support. Some versions allow for water births (exactly like it sounds). Your partner may like the stool as a way to relieve back pressure and move the baby down.

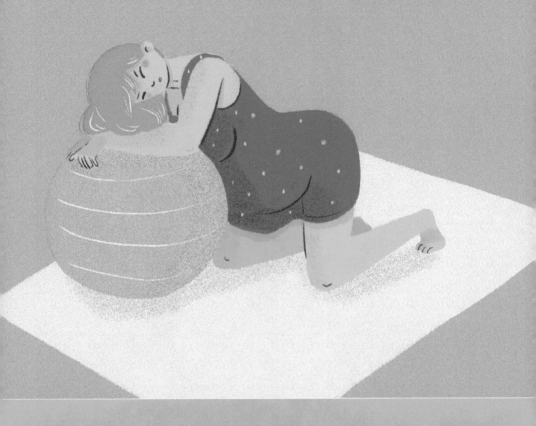

KNEELING BIRTH

She can use this position to help move the baby to the proper position, as the baby should be facing her back. Letting her squeeze your hands as she pushes while kneeling can also ease contraction pain.

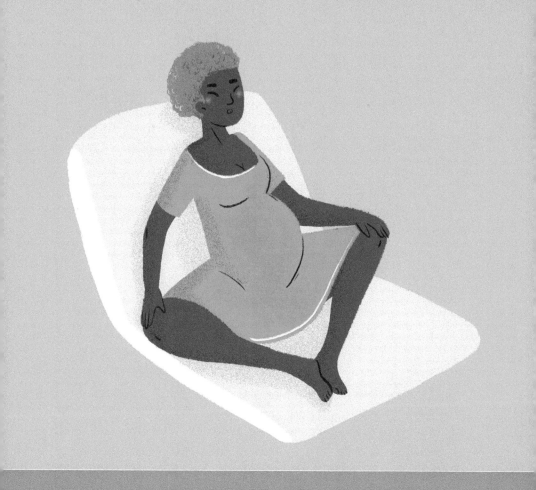

RECLINING

This is what you likely imagine when you're thinking of delivery. She'll get the benefits of relaxed muscles and a break if she's tired from other positions. On the flip side, you lose the effect of gravity. If she chooses this position, see if you can wrap your arm around her thigh so she can push against you.

DELIVERY

It's time to push. Her contractions are frequent and intense. If unmedicated, she'll say she feels like she needs to push, too. Her body will tell her, and it's important that she listens—and that you listen to her.

This is a good time to point out that if you don't think you want to be in the delivery room, you're missing out on the most amazing thing you will ever see in your life. You can handle it. You won't pass out or be "grossed out" in the moment. You won't even think about it. You can stay up by her face the entire time if you'd like. (She may prefer it, anyway.)

If you do nothing else throughout this entire experience, make sure you're a steady-as-a-rock presence when it's time for her to push. In most vaginal deliveries, the baby will be coming out little by little, then all at once. My son started poking out, and then he slipped out like a fish. It was insane.

This stage can take about 30 minutes to an hour, but don't be surprised if it happens quickly. It'll be a blur to you both in hindsight. You are entirely focused on being the best supporter she's ever had for every single minute. You're not texting, you're not thinking through what happens next, and you're not pulling focus. All eyes are on your beautiful, incredible, how-did-I-get-so-lucky-to-know-her partner.

How do you support her? This doesn't have to be overly complicated. She's doing the hardest thing she'll probably ever do in her life. You will be so proud for her. You'll be a little proud of yourself, too.

Assuming she wants you beside her as she pushes, you are there to hold her hand (no, she isn't going to break it) and give her verbal support (which does not involve Bobby Knight–style scream coaching or phrases like "push harder"). In my case, a nurse and I held my wife's hands while we also wrapped an arm around her leg so she could push against us. This all depends on the birthing position.

Are you going to watch the baby come out? Your first response might be "hell no!" However, I suggest you do watch your baby be born.

Why?

For one, most anyone who has witnessed the birth of their child will find it miraculous and mind-boggling. The opportunity may come around only once in a lifetime.

Secondly, when you see the head start popping out—note that it might have a bluish tint—you can report this to mom. It's typically a great motivator that tells her that her efforts are working and there really is a baby in there. She is working so hard because she is desperate to meet this person who formed inside her, the one whose kicks and jabs she has felt. The one she already loves. Some women ask for a mirror for this very reason; they want to see the baby as soon as possible.

Help motivate her to push when the urge comes. Then give her space to rest in between. Be aware that those pushes take a lot of energy and some pushes will be stronger than others. That's fine. Her body is being challenged to stretch and she is working through it bit by bit. Be her advocate if something unexpected happens. You can be the clear thinker to help her review options with the doctor or midwife. No one is expecting you to know all the answers, but as her advocate, your job is to be vocal if the medical team plans to try and do something you know your partner doesn't want. Sometimes, emergencies happen and there's nothing you can do.

In other cases, it can matter. My wife made it clear (and I was ready to speak up for her if she was overwhelmed), that she strongly opposed having a C-section with our twins unless it was absolutely necessary. Her explicit wish gave her doctor the motivation to try for a vaginal birth for a longer period of time. It worked for us. Maybe she still would have needed a C-section if things had played out differently, but at least we would have had our voice heard.

Be her voice.

Be her rock.

She can do this.

IF COMPLICATIONS ARISE

When you see a baby foot hanging out between your wife's legs, you know things are strange. Ideally, the first part of a baby to come out is his or her head.

Remember how I said our twins were born vaginally? It almost didn't happen. My wife very much wanted to avoid a C-section. While a C-section can be the healthiest option for some mothers under certain circumstances, it wasn't our first choice. Since our older child had been a successful vaginal birth, we hoped the same for our twins.

Fortunately, our amazing doctor had no qualms about just reaching up in there and pulling Hannah out by the feet. That's right. My daughter came into the world pulled out by her feet—like you pull a screaming toddler out of a ball pit.

My wife was incredible, especially since the epidural hadn't fully kicked in. (There's a reason I am a big supporter of push presents.) She found extra drive in her reserves that I think pregnant women somehow find—like the turbo boost in *The Fast and the Furious*—and our Hannah came out in no time.

Although no one plans for it, complications can occur. It's useful to have an idea of possible, out-of-the-ordinary, scenarios. Your medical team has plans in place for any of these situations, which can include a recommendation to have a C-section to get your baby out faster. If you're doing a home birth, your midwife will know when a trip to the ER is needed.

Some potential complications:

Umbilical cord problems: Sometimes the cord can get wrapped around the baby's neck, which can cause breathing issues. It may also come out first, called "prolapse," which could cause blood flow issues.

Abnormal heart rate: This can indicate stress on the baby, so the doctor may suggest moving positions. An atypical heart rate is associated with "non-reassuring fetal status." This means the baby isn't thriving and needs increased monitoring and assistance.

Perinatal asphyxia. This refers to a lack of oxygen for your baby, either during labor and delivery or just after birth.

Placenta previa. When the placenta covers the opening of the cervix. In football parlance, it's like a lead blocker who won't get out of the way for the running back.

Shoulder dystocia. Your baby's head is out, but a shoulder is stuck. Ouch.

Excessive bleeding by the mother. A tear in the uterus can cause this, among other issues. This is the most threatening situation for the mom, so do not hesitate to call the doctor if you're doing a home birth.

The list above can be tough to read, but there's no reason to expect the worst. Tens of thousands of babies are born every day. Only a small fraction of women experience complications. I'd be doing a disservice by not acknowledging potential difficulties. So, tuck the information away in your head and keep moving forward, and remember, most of the time we only hear stories about when something goes wrong, not when it goes right.

Yes, You Have Feelings, Too

Obviously, the birth is all about your partner and the baby, but the experience of watching someone you care about go through this can be extremely emotional for you, too. You're about to have a baby. Your life is about to change in every way. So, while the physical nature of childbirth is rightly focused on the mom, the emotional nature of bringing a baby into the world impacts both of you.

You may feel confused, overwhelmed, overjoyed, anxious, and even a little sad that the pregnancy stage is over. My wife was a gorgeous pregnant woman, and there are times I miss that phase of our lives. During delivery, don't expect anyone to ask how you're doing. Take ownership of your emotions. Give yourself a moment to check in, see how you're feeling. This will help when your partner later asks how you felt throughout the whole thing. Staying in touch with your emotions can help you decide if you need to step out for a moment to gather yourself. Pretending this isn't a huge deal for you is not a sign of strength. Your honest communication can set the tone for this new phase of your relationship.

If you're nervous heading into delivery day, ask a guy friend who recently became a father what it felt like on that day. Unfortunately, chances are nobody has asked him. You may not have asked your dad how he handled childbirth either. Talking it out can help.

UNDERSTANDING C-SECTIONS

Quick: What is the most common surgery in the United States?

It's the cesarean section, according to Health.com. One in three US babies is born via C-section; the United States is particularly high in this regard.

Several health and childbirth advocacy organizations, such as the Mayo Clinic and the March of Dimes, emphasize that a C-section is major surgery. When medically necessary, it's a safe, viable solution in difficult circumstances but shouldn't be viewed as a workaround.

Having multiples, for example, doesn't necessarily mean your partner must have a C-section, even if you may find that some doctors assume you will. Yes, it absolutely increases the chances she'll need one, especially if it's more than two (and in that case, godspeed). Even if the first multiple comes out vaginally, the space created can move the other baby (or babies) around and increase the need for a C-section. Regardless of the number of babies you're having at once, it's a good idea to familiarize yourselves with this procedure. Just in case.

In our experience, my wife and I made it clear to our doctor that she wanted to try for a vaginal birth with our twins. She was able to do so, even when our second daughter decided to enter the world feet first (classic second child!). Had we not made that preference clear in our birth plan, we absolutely would have been told that a C-section was the de facto approach.

That's the thing. Labor is all about knowing your options, weighing the pros and cons, and being able to speak to what you want. Your wife has the right to know why a doctor is recommending a procedure. For C-sections, risks can include longer recovery time, increased likelihood of future C-sections, blood clots, trouble breastfeeding, and more. The baby can be affected by the anesthesia and can have an increased likelihood of breathing issues. This explains why "we'll just do a scheduled C-section" should not be a decision you make lightly.

Still, there are legitimate reasons to have one. Many mothers and babies have no issues following the surgery and come away feeling content and grateful for their birth experience. Most important, years later the kids are just fine.

WHAT IS THE C-SECTION PROCEDURE LIKE?

Depending on the situation, your partner could be placed under general anesthesia or remain conscious and receive an epidural instead.

If your partner is awake, she'll feel only pressure as an incision is made and the baby is extracted.

In most cases, you can be in the room for all of this, holding her hand and offering support. Your partner can also ask to witness the baby being born.

The doctor cuts through the skin (sometimes in a "bikini cut") and eventually makes an incision in the uterus.

The baby is born, removed from the mother, and the umbilical cord is cut. You may be the first to hold your newborn, so be ready.

The mother is stitched back up. Talk to her in advance about whether she wants you to stay with the baby while she is taken care of; I'd bet she'd love for you never to leave your baby's side.

If your partner is placed under general anesthesia, it could take several minutes or an hour or more for her to regain consciousness after the birth, which is all the more reason for you to be ready to hold the baby while everyone awaits mom's return to the waking world.

Recovery can last several weeks. Remember, this is major surgery, and she'll be trying to breastfeed (or deal with formula) and be a mom on top of all that.

Be the most patient you have ever been in your entire life, and then more patient on top of that.

When your partner was growing up and imagining having a baby, a C-section was probably not part of that dream. Many moms expect to have a vaginal birth and can feel like they let themselves and their baby down by not doing it that way. But emergencies and complications happen and flexibility with the birth plan is crucial in this case.

If vaginal birth proves elusive, you can be there to remind your partner that this is simply the first day of a long and happy motherhood. You can help her count her blessings—obviously, a healthy baby is a huge blessing—rather than focusing on how the birth could have been more "perfect."

The March of Dimes puts it best: "Remember that having a healthy baby is more important than how the baby is born."

"IT AIN'T OVER TILL IT'S OVER"

This may blow your mind, but did you know that your partner has to deliver *twice*?

The baby is delivered first. Then a pizza.

No, but that would be amazing.

After the baby arrives, the mother hits the third stage of labor—delivery of the placenta. It's the life-giving organ that has fed your baby all this time. Getting the placenta out quickly is crucial to avoid infection and other issues, but it's much less intense than what you just experienced. This process can take a few minutes or more, with lighter contractions. You may even ask to see (or keep) the nutrient-filled placenta after it comes out. It can be fascinating to view what her body created to grow and sustain a human life for nine months.

Take this time for skin-to-skin (sometimes called "kangaroo") contact, in which you take your shirt off and lay the baby on your chest. This is an amazing bonding time as the newborn senses your warmth and heartbeat. Touch is one of the best ways a new dad can connect with this little being. Relax with your baby in between feedings. Take mental note of his or her tiny hands and feet. For preemies, kangaroo care is used to help regulate body temperature and heartbeat. Isn't that amazing? What you do as a dad already matters. Nothing is manlier than a dude doing skin-to-skin with his newborn.

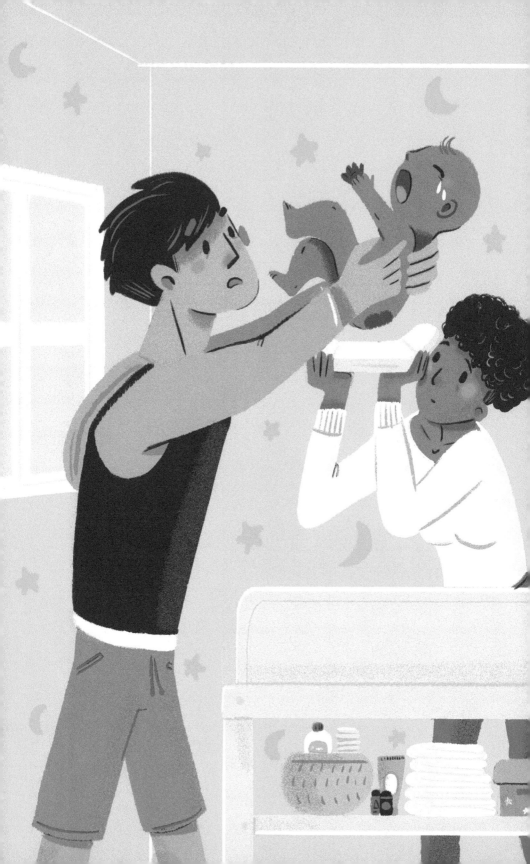

CHAPTER FOUR

IT'S A BABY! NOW WHAT?!

Congratulations! You have a beautiful new baby. This is a monumental, once-in-a-lifetime moment. Even if you have more kids, it'll never be just like this. You helped to create a human being. I made three myself (well, with my wife's help), and I can't even cook dinner.

You'll have plenty of time to dream about your baby's future and worry about how to raise them. That's tomorrow's problem. Today, man . . . today is about relishing what you both have done. Your partner is incredible. I know I gained a deeper appreciation for my wife, Sara, after watching her give birth twice. And by appreciation, I mean: "Holy #%&*! How are you even DOING that?!" And you? You pulled through when she needed you.

Maybe everything wasn't picture perfect. It never is. Maybe your birth plan was ultimately thrown out the window. What matters is what you are now—a family. You are a dad, which means you can now pull off those bad puns and wear all the white Velcro sneakers you want. More important, you're a father that has someone who relies entirely on you to keep them safe and healthy.

Guess what? You can do it, starting from that very first hour.

FATHER OF THE (FIRST) HOUR

Before you get to enjoy your baby, a bunch of medical stuff has to happen. First off, your kiddo is still attached! The umbilical cord has been your baby's lifeline, but now it needs to be cut. And you can be the person to do it.

Don't worry—you can't mess up cutting a cord with what amounts to a pair of safety scissors. Try this scenario to practice: Grab a piece of rope and throw some jelly on it. Glue one end to your dog. Tie the other end to your wife. Now grab the rope and cut it. Did she die? Did you accidentally cut off your dog's tail? Did you get distracted and eat the jelly? If so, cord cutting may not be for you. Also, do not actually tie a rope to your partner.

If you plan to cut the cord, the nurse or doctor will hold the umbilical cord taut after it is clamped and hand you medical scissors. The umbilical cord does not have nerves, so cutting it won't hurt anyone. Some couples wait a few minutes to cut the cord after delivery, to maximize the nutrients going to the baby. This is called delayed cord clamping. You do you.

One snip and you are done. The whole thing takes one second, and it does not impact the way your baby's belly button is shaped. It's a cool dad thing to do. In case you are wondering, the cord feels a bit rubbery and can be slick. But there's no medical reason to have the doctor do it. After all, this is one tiny piece of the delivery process you can truly own. For a few weeks, a little black-ish stump will remain on the belly button, but it will fall off with time.

If she's up for it, you may have a moment here to grab a photo of mom and baby together. She will look so beautiful with that new-mom glow, but give her a minute if she wants one. She might want to put herself together because she knows this photo might show up everywhere. Take lots of photos, but don't be annoying. Take video to look back on years from now. Ask her what she's feeling. She'll probably appreciate that you captured that moment. Get in a photo, too. We had a nurse who was willing to do that for us after delivery was over.

Don't send out the photo unless your partner is ready for the news to be released. She could just want you to let family know everyone is healthy and doing well and maybe the height and weight of the baby. She may want to wait to announce the name if you haven't told anyone that yet. Defer to her on this one. She's waited years for this moment.

By the way, people will ask you the height and weight all the time. It's what people know to ask, and no matter what weight you say, they will have an opinion or compare it to how big their kid was. Or they'll say, "Wow, that's a big boy!" or "Such a tiny angel!" or something like this. They're just trying to make conversation. Keep it funny.

Soon after birth, your baby will face the first of many tests. Early testing helps doctors get a head start, just in case there's anything unusual that pops up.

The baby gets an Apgar score, which checks for: Appearance, Pulse, Grimace, Activity, and Respiration. Essentially, they are making sure the baby is breathing properly, responding to stimuli, and has a good blood flow.

This test happens right away—you can be beside your newborn during it all—and if the score is low, some suctioning of the airway or additional measures to give your baby a little extra help may be required.

Once all this is done, you'll get to a recovery room, but more tests are on the way.

You have the right to be there for any tests. As the dad, you may be better situated to do this while your partner is recovering. Do *not* assume any of these tests mean doctors are concerned. It's protocol. It's their first chance to assess your baby outside of the belly.

Here's what your baby may be tested and screened for:

Blood test: Your newborn will be screened for a variety of metabolic, genetic, and endocrine disorders. This involves a quick heel prick to get a few drops of blood. I know you or your partner may not love the idea of your brand-spanking-new baby getting a needle already, but it's important. Your kid is not going to hold this against you years from now. Results come back within a week. If there's something that gets flagged, it may mean additional tests.

Pulse oximetry: This test checks the oxygen level in the blood, which can indicate a heart issue if it's low. There is no pain with this procedure.

Hearing test: There are two options for this. In one version, a soft earphone and microphone are placed in the ear. The earphone plays sounds, and the microphone measures the ear's response. In the other, soft earphones are placed in the ears. Electrodes on your baby's head measure how her auditory nerve and brain stem respond.

State requirements vary, and you can also request additional tests. These may or may not be covered by insurance if there is a genetic history or other reasons to screen.

MOTHER OF THE (FIRST) HOUR

Keep in mind that the mom's recovery experience varies depending on whether she had natural childbirth or a C-section, as well as other factors (fitness level, preexisting conditions, and more can impact recovery rate). Her doctor or midwife will talk with her about what to expect as well as potential emotional changes, as there will be plenty of hormones affecting her recovery. You can be supportive by making sure she has her favorite meals, toiletries, and other comforting items. If you detect a prolonged, depressed mood change, support her decision to see a doctor. It's better to be cautious.

After delivery is finished, the mother's uterus should start to return to normal size. It is normal for her to still "look pregnant" for a period of time after the birth. This can be a tough mental hurdle for her because of society's pressure for women to snap back into their pre-baby shape quickly. That's not how bodies work.

At this point, you have experienced childbirth—vaginal or C-section. You witnessed the pain, the struggle, and felt the overwhelming joy. You have already done so much to support your partner and baby. However, if you think it all ends just because she leaves the hospital, you might want to update your sensitivity chip.

Long after you cut off your hospital band, your partner's body is trying to piece itself back together. Keep this in mind when you approach the new mom. This can be an extra-sensitive time for most mothers, and it's always wise to think before you speak. It can take a new mother up to a year to recover from childbirth, especially if a C-section is involved. In the meantime, she's dealing with:

Vaginal soreness. Did you know she can get brush burns on her vagina from birth? Have you ever had a brush burn? Has it been on your vagina? If the answer is yes, then I have a whole new set of questions for you. Otherwise, take it from my wife; it's very painful.

Perineal tear. Essentially, this is a tear beneath her vagina which can require stitches. Sometimes the tear is created via an episiotomy, a cut made into her perineum to enlarge the vaginal opening. Obviously, this is uncomfortable at best. She may require checkups to make sure the wound is healing properly.

Afterpains (post-childbirth contractions). These can take up to six to eight weeks to shrink the uterus back to size. This is not like deflating a balloon. It's like squeezing Silly Putty into a smaller container.

Breast engorgement. Regardless of your personal views on breast size and shape, milk-swollen breasts *do not* feel awesome. As her breasts fill up with milk, they can harden and hurt. Warm compresses and massage while pumping or feeding can help. You'll hear women say it feels like their boobs are going to explode. This is also why they say "look but don't touch."

Mastitis. This is an inflammation of breast tissue that can cause swelling, redness, and pain. It's common, and it's painful. Mastitis happens because of a clogged milk duct. A cold compress can help.

Nipple soreness. If she's breastfeeding, her nipples feel like they are on the wrong end of a *Game of Thrones* wedding. The skin may sting, crack, and bleed. Do not hesitate to call on a lactation consultant or doula to help with the pain or the baby's latch.

Empathy is your friend here, especially because everyone will focus on the baby. They may forget that your partner just gave birth, so it's your job to remember. From her crown chakra to the tip of her toes, every part of her body has been through the ringer. Be gentle, patient, and curious when she lets you know how she's feeling. She's probably completely exhausted. If it's her first child, she may not yet understand the ever-changing tides that her body, hormones, and mind are experiencing.

If you can offer a regular massage, do it. If you're terrible at massages and can afford to send her for one, do it. Postpartum massages can be wonderful.

If the best you can do is ask if you can buy her some Tylenol and a heat wrap at the pharmacy, do that. Just don't let it be something you forget about because she definitely can't.

You and your partner just participated in a miracle.

That first day will fly by. Appreciate all that was accomplished. It's incredible. If even for a moment, you are holding the newest human being in the entire world. And that baby is yours. Bravo!

GETTING YOUR DAD ROLE DOWN ON DAY ONE

It's a thrill to have your baby at home that first full day.

The joy—and apprehension—can send a chill up your spine.

Thrills and chills—and, probably, some spills—are all parts of bringing home baby. It's a vortex of emotions and activity, but you can do this. What may strike you first is the distinct lack of support. At the hospital, there are nurses to take the baby when mom is tired and to help at every feeding, every diaper change, and every temperature check. There was the secure feeling of having a doctor on staff in case something felt wrong. Now it's just you and your partner. (And, if you're lucky, a trusted granny.)

Remember to take a deep breath. Your partner is probably also freaking out, even if it's on the inside. Now is the time to get into dad mode. Don't take on any new projects like organizing photos on your iPhone. Your baby needs you. Your partner needs you. They don't need you to be perfect. But they need you to be present and try your best, even if all you can do is change a diaper or practice your swaddle.

Bathing

The baby's first bath won't be in your tub. You can simply use a basin with warm water—never hot—mild soap, and a soft washcloth. Start with the face and work your way down, leaving genitals for last. Make sure to wash easy-to-miss areas like behind the ears and in between skin folds. You or your partner can hold your baby the entire time; it's a fun bonding experience to have both of you involved.

Be careful to monitor your baby's breathing and make sure they don't get cold; remember, they were just inside a cozy belly for many months. The umbilical cord stump is still going to be there for another week or two—resist the urge to pull on it. It'll fall off when it is meant to.

Once you're done, pat baby to dry off. Put a diaper on the baby right away or you may regret it. Baby boys can turn into sprinklers when the warm water hits them. Baby powder is no longer recommended by many doctors since the fine powder can get into a baby's lungs. Just make sure you dry off their genital area, and if there is a rash, use a diaper cream.

Feeding

Some moms will breastfeed with no issue. Others will be able to do it, but only after considerable effort and struggle. For many moms, it doesn't work out at all. There is no "right" approach as long as your baby is healthy. Your role is to help mom feel as supported as possible. Breastfeeding can be fraught with tons of emotional baggage, physical hurdles, and stigma. ("Are you nursing?" is a common question moms face, and there always seems to be some kind of hidden agenda behind it.) Be patient. Be understanding. Make sure she has something to drink and a comfortable spot. Buy her some extra nursing bras (which unhook differently) if she wants, as she'll be wearing them nonstop. Read up on her rights to nurse in public, and advocate for her when she needs you to. It may be possible for your partner to request a visit from a lactation consultant, a specialist who focuses on helping moms with breastfeeding.

Most hospitals will highly encourage at least a few days of breastfeeding, if possible. If formula is the route you end up taking at some point, you can help warm the bottle and prepare everything, especially in the middle of the night. You can also help her track feedings and how much the baby ate.

Bottle Duty

Cleaning baby bottles can be a great way to help. It's smart to use a separate counter mat and sponge to reduce cross-contamination. If your wife nurses, she may have a breast pump, which has its own set of parts to clean.

Diapers

Dads should take on diaper duty—you are not "pitching in" or "helping." This is your job. Movies often depict dads deferring to the mothers to take on a poopy diaper as though she is obligated to take the reins on every aspect of child care. Take charge of keeping all the diaper changing areas and bags stocked with diapers and wipes (try the hypoallergenic options, as baby skin is prone to rashes). In cold climates, some parents swear by wipe warmers. Some parents find they are overkill. Be sure to stock your dude diaper bag with a mat you can roll out when you have to do a change on the road. You don't want to be left in some random gas station that doesn't have a clean baby changing table. Even today, many men's restrooms don't have one. Oh, and take on emptying the Diaper Genie. It's disgusting, yes, but it builds character. No? Clean it anyway.

Swaddling

Your childbirth class likely covered this, but mastering the art of the swaddle makes you that much more useful. Swaddling helps a baby feel secure, like they are back in the womb. (Seriously, most of keeping a baby happy is making them feel like they are in the womb. That's why white noise machines can work wonders at night.) There are Velcro versions to simplify things if you don't want to try the muslin cloth route. You can swaddle until the baby learns to roll over, but that won't be for months.

Nap Time/Bedtime

Putting my kids down for bed is one of the most challenging yet rewarding things I've done as a dad. I tried to take ownership of it early on because it gave my wife time to herself right after breastfeeding.

Some baby experts recommend that new parents avoid getting in the habit of rocking the baby. On the contrary, many grandmothers say a good rocking chair will be your best friend. I agree with the grandmothers. Rock and sing to your baby, even if your voice is terrible. Read to them. Tell them a story. Whatever it is, the baby wants to hear your voice and will start to identify your voice with a calming sensation.

When you get the baby to sleep, gently place her on her back—always on her back—in a crib or on a similar flat surface. If he or she starts to cry, you can try gently patting or talking to him or her. The latest research shows that the crib should not have pillows, loose blankets, or even crib bumpers—nothing that can cause suffocation. Don't assume that just because it's in a store it's safe. Your baby just needs a firm, flat mattress.

When you're running on adrenaline during those first few days, you may find yourself falling asleep in a recliner with your newborn. The photos may be cute, but it's actually quite dangerous. Don't try it. If you are holding the baby and think you may fall asleep, either have someone else on alert or hand off the baby. It's not worth the risk.

Bonding

Try kangaroo care! Take off your shirt and place your baby (in just a diaper) on your chest. They will soak up your body heat, sense your heartbeat, and love the closeness. It's an awesome way to bond, and you have an advantage as a dad. With mom, the baby might feel like it's feeding time, but you can just enjoy the closeness.

Dealing with Crying or Colic

One of the things that might change most in your household those first few days is the sound. It might feel like you don't remember what it sounded like before you had a baby. Although I've heard stories of magical newborns who sleep all the time, most babies "wake up" a few hours or a few days after coming home. A newborn can get loud, and the constant crying can be nerve-racking. Prepare yourself ahead of time, know it won't last forever, and be patient. Tap into that newfound love that you never even knew existed and find ways to calm them down slowly. Newborns are usually either tired, hungry, or overstimulated. Taking them for a walk in a stroller, a car ride, or just rocking them can do the trick. Or not. Just keep calm and keep trying.

If your baby cries for long periods and doesn't respond to comforting measures like being taken for a walk or held close to your body, your baby may be experiencing colic. Colic is prolonged, unexplained crying in an otherwise healthy infant. Some families find relief for colic by offering infant massage, learning how to swaddle the baby, or by changing the mother's diet to remove common allergens that could be affecting the baby. If your baby is experiencing colic, discuss with our midwife or pediatrician to begin exploring what may help your baby feel calm and content. Remember that while colic can be stressful and upsetting, many babies experience it and go on to be happy and healthy. Be patient and work with your partner to support each other if you feel frazzled or distressed by your baby's crying. Take deep breaths or go for some walks by yourself. Above all, know that this too shall pass.

GETTING INTO THE SWING OF THINGS

Two things will become quickly apparent in those first few days. One, your baby craves a routine. Babies feel like they have no control over anything; after all, they would have preferred to stay in the womb. Whatever you can do to give them a routine can help. For example, you can start a consistent process of taking the baby from your partner after she feeds. Then it's time for a diaper change and a swaddle before you rock them to sleep or go for a walk. A schedule will ultimately help the whole household.

My wife and I erred by not giving our son a consistent nap time. To this day, we kick ourselves over our naive thought that we would let him decide when he was tired. Instead, all we got was a baby who had no idea when to expect to nap, and he never learned.

The other apparent truth is that your own routine won't exist. It all tends to circle around what your baby needs at first, and with good reason. They can't do anything for themselves yet. Even if you're back to work, your nightly routine won't be the same. A fever, a fussy night, or trouble feeding can all throw things off. You have an important role in being flexible and understanding that this too shall pass. Your partner is likely doing everything she can just to have a shred of normalcy (on top of physically recovering). It will do you no good to complain about not being able to do something that's your usual thing at the usual time.

Instead, see what you can do to keep checking items off the list. Not only is that part of your duty as the dad, it's the fast track to the two of you finding your own time to be together. If bottles are dirty, the laundry is piling up, and insurance billing is left unresolved, your partner is not going to relax. Control what you can control, and know that the rest will find its own rhythm soon enough.

If the lack of consistency is getting to you, don't keep it inside. Talk with your partner as it comes. Don't bottle it up and end up venting your frustration in unhelpful ways. Remember that she may not be able to solve anything, but at least she'll know where you're coming from.

Recovery Partner

Your mission as a rock-solid partner doesn't end just because the baby has arrived. In fact, some women may have a harder time after birth, especially emotionally. It's important that you don't chalk everything up to hormones or downplay it if she says she's having a tough time.

Physically, new moms can face issues such as exhaustion, bleeding, bladder control problems, breast tenderness, and more. Support her by grabbing ice packs, pain medication, or taking the baby for a ride while she naps or sleeps in for a bit. Whatever else she needs, a post-birth doctor visit can help address these, too.

Communicating with your partner about her emotions and the "baby blues" is important. Postpartum depression or anxiety is much more than just feeling down. A new mother may feel disconnected or apathetic about her baby. She may have anxiety about the baby's well-being to the point that she can't sleep. If you feel like your partner is having more than just a few rough days, talk with her about how she's feeling. Postpartum mental health issues are not uncommon, and she's not less of a mom for having them. Even if she appears fine for the first few weeks or months, be aware that postpartum depression or anxiety can begin at any time in the first year. Treatment options are available.

Being a new parent can feel overwhelming in between the joyful moments. The lack of sleep doesn't help. You are not obligated to entertain guests or say yes to every visitor request. You need to prioritize mom and baby, and avoid germs, too. Be a buffer for them. Let people know that you'll be ready to accept visitors in a few weeks or ask if they could instead run an errand for you. Good friends will understand.

AND OFF YOU GO

Throughout all of this, you're going to be tested. Being a parent refines your character. I'm a better person as a dad than I was before, and that's in part to all the early tests I faced. Some days, I crushed it. I felt like Super Dad. And others? Man, I wish I had a do-over.

What won't work for either of you is focusing on how the other person approaches parenthood. Both of you are figuring it out. The only thing that matters is raising a healthy and happy kid. If she decides to do something differently than you would, but there's no harm done, let it go. It's not worth fighting over.

Figure out early on what, if anything, is nonnegotiable. It's easier to let the other person know where the line is before they accidentally cross it. For us, we didn't want to fall asleep holding our son because of the danger factor. So, if my wife woke me up and said, "Hey, you really need to watch that," I knew she wasn't mad at me—she was protecting all of us. Know the difference. This isn't the time to take things personally, and it's not the time to find flaws. You both need each other, and that's what's going to make you amazing parents.

All of this can feel like a lot to consume and remember. You are more capable of being a remarkable involved father than you know. Nobody starts out in the All-Star Dad League. Even if their Instagram profile is full of nothing but magazine-worthy moments, rest assured they've had their share of setbacks, failures, and gray-hair inducing nights. Fatherhood is what happens in between all the pictures.

Take a deep breath and realize that if you forget everything else, all you need to do is support your partner and your baby in a way that makes them feel loved. You can definitely do this, and your newly expanded family believes in you, too.

Resources

The New Mom's Guide to New Dads
Give your partner a boost of confidence with my book that focuses on helping her understand what you're going through. There are even a few chapters dedicated to new dads! See more at Instafather.com.

Parenting.NYTimes.com
This is broken down by life stages and is chock-full of researched-based stories and guides.

Dad2.com/blog
A national organization, Dad 2.0 has evolved from a summit for dad bloggers into a platform for fatherhood.

WebMD.com/pregnancy-app
There's a contraction timer, visualizations of your unborn baby week-by-week, and science-backed research.

LLLI.org
La Leche League International can be a great source of breast-feeding support and knowledge for both of you should your partner decide to breastfeed.

References

American Pregnancy Association. "Patterned Breathing During Labor: Techniques and Benefits." Accessed March 2020. AmericanPregnancy.org/labor-and-birth/patterned-breathing.

American Pregnancy Association. "Stages of Labor." Accessed April 2020. AmericanPregnancy.org/labor-and-birth/what-is -the-first-stage-of-labor.

CDC. "Reproductive Health: Premature Birth." Accessed March 2020. www.CDC.gov/reproductivehealth/features/premature-birth /index.html.

Childbirth Connection. "Labor Induction Basics." Accessed April 2020. ChildbirthConnection.org/giving-birth /labor-induction/basics.

Childbirth Connection. "Report of the Third National U.S. Survey of Women's Childbearing Experiences." Published May 2013. NationalPartnership.org/our-work/resources/health-care /maternity/listening-to-mothers-iii-major-findings.pdf.

Decker, Rebecca. "Breathing for pain relief during labor." Published August 7, 2018. EvidenceBasedBirth.com/breathing-for-pain -relief-during-labor.

Gerber Baby Blog. "What Is a Receiving Blanket?" Accessed April 2020. GerberChildrensWear.com/blogs/news/what-is-a -receiving-blanket.

Greenhalgh, Jane. "To Reduce Infant Deaths, Doctors Call For A Ban Of Crib Bumpers." Published November 25, 2015. NPR.org/sections/health-shots/2015/11/25/457285189/to -reduce-infant-deaths-doctors-call-for-a-ban-of-crib-bumpers.

Grow By WebMD. "Normal Labor and Delivery Process." Accessed April 2020. WebMD.com/baby/guide/normal-labor-and -delivery-process#1.

Grow By WebMD. "Understanding Preterm Labor and Birth— Diagnosis and Treatment." Accessed April 2020. WebMD .com/baby/magnesium-sulfate-for-preterm-labor.

Healthline Parenthood. "Lamaze Breathing." Accessed April 2020. Healthline.com/health/lamaze-breathing#the-lamaze -method.

Huizen, Jennifer. "What to Know About Membrane Stripping." Published August 8, 2018. MedicalNewsToday.com /articles/322701#is-it-effective.

Kaiser Permanente. "Your Pregnancy: Weeks 37 to 40." Accessed March 2020. Healthy.KaiserPermanente.org/health-wellness /maternity/third-trimester/weeks-37-40.

Levine, Hallie. "Home Birth Is Growing in Popularity. Is It Right for You?" Published April 18, 2020. Parenting.NYTimes.com /pregnancy/home-birth.

March of Dimes. "Newborn Screening Tests for Your Baby." Accessed April 202. MarchofDimes.org/baby/newborn -screening-tests-for-your-baby.aspx#.

Marcin, Ashley. "What Do Braxton-Hicks Feel Like." Published August 22, 2019. Healthline.com/health/parenting/what -do-braxton-hicks-feel-like.

Marple, Kate. "How Big Is My Baby?" Accessed March 2020. BabyCenter.com/slideshow-baby-size.

Mayo Clinic. "Home birth: Know the Pros and Cons." Accessed April 2020. MayoClinic.org/healthy-lifestyle/labor-and -delivery/in-depth/home-birth/art-20046878.

Mayo Clinic. "Labor and Deliver, Postpartum Care." Accessed April 2020. MayoClinic.org/healthy-lifestyle/labor-and -delivery/in-depth/labor-and-delivery/art-2004936.

Mayo Clinic. "Labor Induction." Accessed April 2020. MayoClinic. org/tests-procedures/labor-induction/about /pac-20385141.

Mayo Clinic. "Pregnancy Week by Week." Accessed February 2020. www.mayoclinic.org/healthy-lifestyle/pregnancy-week-by -week/in-depth/fetal-development/art-20045997.

Mazel, Sharon. "Labor Positions." Last modified May 12, 2020. WhatToExpect.com/pregnancy/labor-and-delivery /delivery-options/labor-positions.aspx.

Migala, Jessica. "Beyoncé Reveals She Had an Emergency Section. Here's What the Procedure Really Does to Your Body." Published August 6, 2018. Health.com/condition/pregnancy/c-section.

Murray, Linda. "Newborn screening tests: Which ones your baby will have and why." Published August 31, 2019. BabyCenter .com/0_newborn-screening-tests-which-ones-your-baby-will -have-and-w_1471069.bc.

Pampers Blog. "8 Months Pregnant: Symptoms and Fetal Development." Accessed March 2020. Pampers.com/en-us /pregnancy/pregnancy-calendar/8-months-pregnant.

Smith, Lori. "Ten Common Labor Complications." Last modified June 27, 2018. MedicalNewsToday.com/articles/307462.

U.S. Department of Health & Human Services - Women's Health. "Stages of Pregnancy." Accessed March 2020. WomensHealth.gov/pregnancy/youre-pregnant-now-what /stages-pregnancy.

Waldron, Patricia. "What to Expect During the Three Stages of Labor." Last modified April 18, 2020. Parenting.NYTimes.com /pregnancy/signs-of-labor.

Index

F

Fatigue, 8
Feeding, 76. *See also* Breastfeeding
Feelings and emotions, 23–24, 64, 81
Fetal heart monitoring, 15
"5-1-1" rule for contractions, 41–42
Full term, 1

G

Group B streptococcus (GBS) test, 15

H

Hands and knees position, 53
Hearing test, 72
Hemorrhoids, 7
Home births, 11–12
Hormones, 28, 72
Hospital bags, 24–27
Hospitals, 9–12

I

Induction, 37–39
Insurance, 11–12, 27

K

Kangaroo care, 10–11, 67, 78
Kneeling position, 52, 58

L

Labor
active, 33, 41–43
early, 32–34
positions, 47–55, 56–59
signs of, 30–32
transition stage, 33, 43–44
Labor augmentation, 5
Lactation support, 10
Lamaze, 13, 55
Leaning over position, 52
Lightening, 31
Lotions, 25

M

Mastitis, 73
Maternity gowns, 24
Medical tests, 14–15, 71–72
Membrane stripping/ sweeping, 38
Midwives, 10, 12
Music, 25

N

Nap time, 77–78
Neonatal intensive care units (NICUs), 19–20
Ninth month, 28–29
Nipple soreness, 74
Nonstress test, 15

About the Author

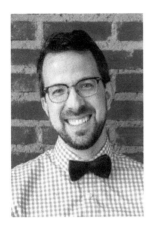

Andrew Shaw is an award-winning parenting columnist, former journalist, and creator of *InstaFather*, a blog dedicated to helping new parents, especially dads. He is a married, Pennsylvania-born father of three (a son and twin girls). In between constantly getting these kids snacks, he's a marketing strategist and a professional improv comedian who has toured across the mid-Atlantic. Andrew's work has been featured on *Scary Mommy, The Good Men Project, Fatherly,* and *Central Penn Parent.* He's also the author of *The New Mom's Guide to New Dads* (2020).

CPSIA information can be obtained
at www.ICGtesting.com
Printed in the USA
JSHW051047210820
7391JS00005B/1